KT-414-550

Clinicians' Guide to Growth Disorders

Clinicians' Guide to Growth Disorders

J. K. H. Wales
DM, MA, BM, BCh, FRCPCH, MRCP
Senior Lecturer in Paediatric Endocrinology, University of Sheffield,
Sheffield Children's Hospital, Sheffield, UK

A member of the Hodder Headline Group
LONDON   NEW YORK   NEW DELHI

First published in Great Britain in 2002 by
Arnold, a member of the Hodder Headline Group,
338 Euston Road, London NW1 3BH

http://www.arnoldpublishers.com

Distributed in the United States of America by
Oxford University Press Inc.,
198 Madison Avenue, New York, NY10016
Oxford is a registered trademark of Oxford University Press

© 2002 J. K. H. Wales

All rights reserved. No part of this publication may be reproduced or transmitted in any
form or by any means, electronically or mechanically, including photocopying, recording or
any information storage or retrieval system, without either prior permission in writing from
the publisher or a licence permitting restricted copying. In the United Kingdom such
licences are issued by the Copyright Licensing Agency: 90 Tottenham Court Road,
London W1P 0LP

Whilst the advice and information in this book are believed to be true and accurate at the
date of going to press, neither the author nor the publisher can accept any legal
responsibility or liability for any errors or omissions that may be made. In particular (but
without limiting the generality of the preceding disclaimer) every effort has been made to
check drug dosages; however it is still possible that errors have been missed. Furthermore,
dosage schedules are constantly being revised and new side-effects recognized. For these
reasons the reader is strongly urged to consult the drug companies' printed instructions
before administering any of the drugs recommended in this book.

British Library Cataloguing in Publication Data
A catalogue record for this book is available from the British Library

Library of Congress Cataloging-in-Publication Data
A catalog record for this book is available from the Library of Congress

ISBN 0 340 76237 3

1 2 3 4 5 6 7 8 9 10

Commissioning Editor: Nick Dunton
Production Editor: Rada Radojicic
Production Controller: Bryan Eccleshall

Typeset in 11/13pt Adobe Garamond by Phoenix Photosetting, Chatham, Kent
Printed and bound in Malta by Gutenberg Press

What do you think about this book? Or any other Arnold title?
Please send your comments to feedback.arnold@hodder.co.uk

Contents

Preface

This book is designed to give a comprehensive account of growth disorders in children for the primary care physician and the 'paediatrician with an interest', as well as for paediatricians in training, auxologists, health workers or interested medical students.

The measurement of growth is a simple procedure that is often performed very badly. Individuals need training in technique and data plotting, and the standards used for comparison must be current. When performed correctly, growth monitoring is a useful non-invasive tool for the assessment of the health and psychosocial environment of a child. Although unselected growth screening of the population is of little value, for the individual child presenting in primary care measurement of height and weight should be just as routine a part of clinical assessment as taking their temperature. Such measurement should always be undertaken in any child about whom there is parental or professional concern.

Many pathologies affect growth, and a careful examination and assessment of pubertal status may often reveal a cause. Systemic disorders may render a child short and thin, whereas most endocrine disorders result in a short child who is relatively overweight. Syndromic short stature is surprisingly common, and some causes of disproportionate short stature are now amenable to treatment. Delayed puberty is a common cause of concern to both child and parent, and is usually easy to diagnose and treat. Although they present less often for assessment, pathologies that result in tall stature are important. Early sexual development is very common, mainly due to variations of normality or secondary to obesity, which itself is rapidly becoming one of the major health problems encountered in paediatrics. Failure to thrive is often non-organic, but may present a challenge to the primary or secondary care team.

Most of the example charts in this book are taken from real examples that have presented to our endocrine clinic.

I think that paediatric endocrinology is the most fascinating and rewarding area of medicine, and I hope that some of my enthusiasm will be transmitted by this book and will inform and stimulate those who care for the health of all children.

I wish to thank Mrs Margaret Pickering, auxologist, without whose records this work would not have been possible and to whom I dedicate this book, and my friend and colleague Dr Neil Wright, for his help and suggestions during the preparation of this text.

J. K. H. Wales

Introduction

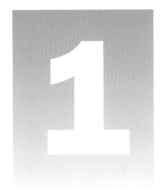

The physiology of growth

Growth at all stages of human development is the end-product of a complex interaction between nutrient supply (over and above that required for basic metabolism) and hormones on the skeleton, with any surplus energy being converted to muscle or deposited as fat. The process is easily disrupted and can serve as a marker for pathologies in any system, as well as in the child's social environment.

There are four phases to human growth, namely fetal, infantile, childhood and pubertal, each of which has different predominating control mechanisms.

Fetal growth

This is the most rapid phase of growth, peaking at 10 cm/month at the end of the second trimester, with maximal weight gain at 34–36 weeks' gestation. Placental nutrient supply is the main constraint on growth. The placenta is also an active endocrine organ that produces growth factors such as growth hormone variant and placental lactogen, as well as organ-specific hormones such as corticotrophin-releasing hormone (CRH), hepatic and epidermal growth factors that act on the adrenal and liver, respectively (see Figure 1.1).

The placenta is a rich source of steroids for both mother and fetus, and it also acts to remove some fetal adrenal steroids. It actively secretes growth factors that affect both the fetus as a whole and also specific organs such as the fetal adrenal and liver. Some maternal thyroxine reaches the fetus in early gestation, and in later gestation the placenta 'deactivates' fetal thyroxine by converting it into an inactive form.

The placenta allows a small amount of thyroxine to pass to the fetus in early pregnancy, and this has important effects on later brain development. Thereafter the placenta is relatively impermeable to thyroxine and deactivates

Figure 1.1
Nutrients for growth are delivered from the mother to the fetus via the placenta.

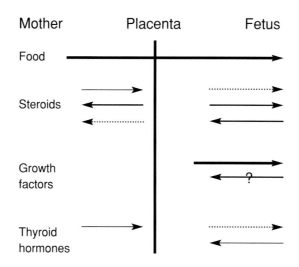

Mother   Placenta   Fetus

Food

Steroids

Growth factors

Thyroid hormones

fetal thyroxine. It acts as a barrier to two-way fetal and maternal steroid production, as well as producing placental steroids that may subsequently affect blood-pressure. The fetal pancreas releases insulin in response to fuel supply, and this has direct growth-promoting effects. In addition, the fetus manufactures insulin-like growth factors 1 and 2 (IGF-1 and IGF-2) and modulates their actions with specific binding proteins.

Box 1.1 Causes of a small baby

Small parents (especially the mother)
Twins, triplets, etc.
Prematurity

Symmetrical IUGR:
- congenital infection
- chromosomal and syndromic abnormalities
- early placental damage/dysfunction – smoking
- extreme starvation, maternal ill health.

Asymmetrical IUGR:
- late placental partial detachment/infarction
- post-maturity
- late nutrient deficiency
- pre-eclampsia.

Inadequate nutrient supply due to placental failure or damage will result in intrauterine growth retardation (IUGR), which may be symmetrical if it occurs early in pregnancy (weight, length and head circumference are all affected), or it may be asymmetrical (with mainly weight affected) if associated with later problems. Premature birth may result in suboptimal growth at a critical phase. Although later catch-up growth is usual, there may be late metabolic consequences (e.g. hypertension, insulin resistance).

Size at birth is therefore much more closely related to the mother's size, nutrition and placental health than to any influence from the father. A large mother married to a small man a or a tall mother with gestational diabetes may produce a large baby who later moves across the centiles to occupy a lower position by 2 years of age. This is a normal phenomenon ('catch-down growth') that is no cause for concern.

Likewise, a small mother may have a small baby who shows catch-up growth in both weight and height centiles postnatally, which should not be misinterpreted as excessive weight gain due to overfeeding. About 60% of IUGR babies will show catch-up growth after removal of any intrauterine constraint, especially those with asymmetrical growth retardation, although 10–30% in various reported series will remain short as adults.

Thus by 2 years of age a child should occupy a height centile that is determined to the same extent by both parents' size, but before then a considerable amount of 'channel-crossing' on the centile charts may occur (see Figure 1.2).

Infantile growth

This is often regarded as an extension of the fetal growth phase (i.e. determined mainly by nutrition) before growth hormone becomes the predominant controller of growth, in the second year of life. An increase in height and weight requires adequate nutrition but also a normally functioning thyroid gland and normal bone mineralization. The hypothalamic–pituitary axis is increasingly important, and children with growth hormone deficiency are shorter than might be expected even during the first year.

Most concerns at this age relate to failure to gain weight at an adequate rate (failure to thrive (FTT); see Chapter 7). If poor weight gain is prolonged, there will be a subsequent faltering of length and then head circumference.

Childhood growth

Growth in height requires the action of growth hormone (GH) on epiphyseal cartilage cells to produce IGF-1, the major postnatal growth factor,

GIRLS PRE-TERM (30wks gestation) - 52 WEEKS

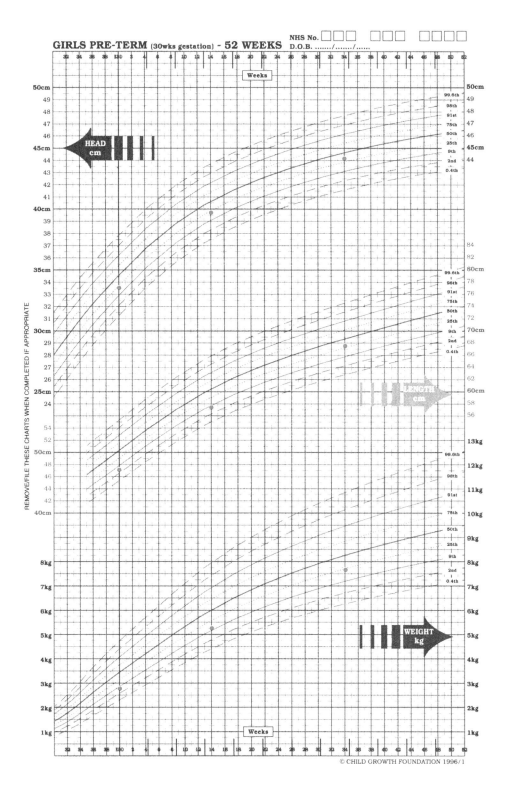

REMOVE/FILE THESE CHARTS WHEN COMPLETED IF APPROPRIATE

© CHILD GROWTH FOUNDATION 1996/1

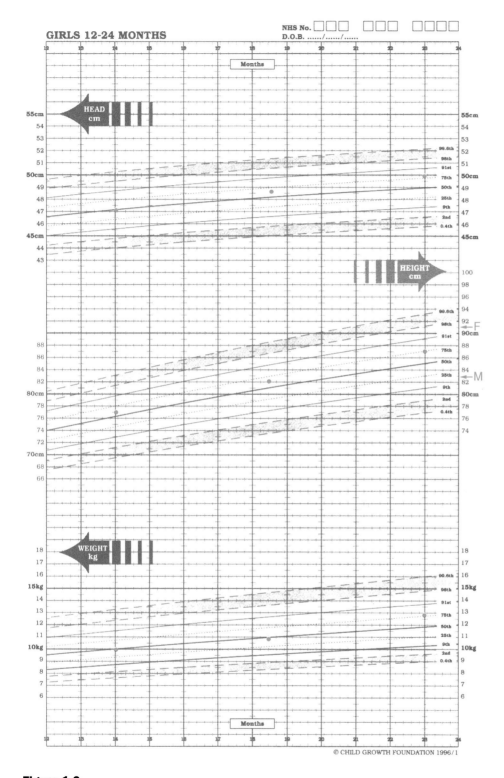

Figure 1.2

Baby girl born on 9th centile, equivalent to mother's (155.5 cm) adult size centile. Tall father (196 cm), equivalent to 99.6th centile. Normal 'catch-up' growth to genetic centile by 2 years of age.

which in turn stimulates cell division and growth. This requires adequate nutrition, a normal skeleton, normal calcium and vitamin D status and euthyroidism.

Growth hormone is a single-chain 191-amino-acid polypeptide which is produced by the anterior pituitary and circulates complexed to a binding protein (GHBP). GH is secreted in an intermittent, pulsatile pattern largely due to the reciprocal interactions of two hypothalamic peptides, namely GH-releasing hormone (GHRH) and somatostatin or somatotropin-release-inhibiting factor (SRIF). In addition to growth hormone itself there are a number of peptides (e.g. IGF-I) and neurotransmitters that control GH release which can be modulated by input from higher centres, and GH release is therefore maximal in a happy, unstressed child.

The actions of IGF-1 are controlled by binding to several binding proteins (IGFBPs) which may in turn be affected by immune modulators such as cytokines, thus reducing their availability in states of inflammation.

Figure 1.3
Control of GH secretion from higher centres through hypothalamic releasing and inhibitory factors. Circulating GH is bound to a binding protein, and generates IGF-1 in the liver, which then circulates bound to various proteins. IGF-1 is also generated in cartilage for autocrine (same-cell) and paracrine (neighbouring-cell) action. IGF-1 release in the circulation and periphery is controlled by nutritional status, cytokines and proteases. Other factors required are adequate vitamin D, calcium and phosphate intake, normal liver and renal function, oestrogen secretion (or conversion from testosterone by aromatase) and thyroxine.

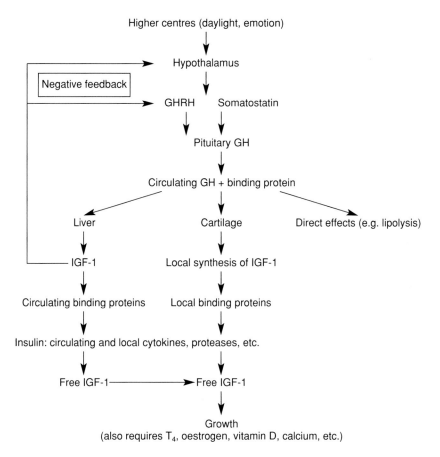

Pubertal growth and final height

At puberty the pulsatile release of GH is increased by two- to threefold, after which the secretion of GH returns towards prepubertal values and then declines from middle age onwards (the 'somatopause').

In addition, the gonads produce the sex hormones testosterone and oestrogen. These act particularly to boost the growth of the spine – hence the long-legged body habitus of a hypogonadotrophic individual with normal GH production (e.g. untreated Klinefelter's syndrome). At the same time, oestrogen (in both sexes – in the male by aromatization in the periphery) acts to mature the epiphyses towards eventual bony fusion, after which growth ceases.

Final size is determined by inheritance from both parents, but the mechanisms underlying this programming of stature are obscure.

With improved nutrition (especially protein and total calorie intake) there is a secular trend towards increasing height, weight and earlier sexual maturation in each generation such that growth standards need to be regularly updated. The current 9 centile (0.4th, 2nd, 9th, 25th, 50th, 75th, 91st, 98th, 99.6th) UK charts were created from 1990 data and published in 1995. They will be further updated about once per decade, and all previous charts should be regarded as obsolete.

Sexual development

The earliest biochemical event of puberty is the appearance of nocturnal peaks of the gonadotropins LH and FSH secondary to pulsatile secretion of gonadotropin-releasing hormone (GnRH) from the hypothalamus. This stimulates the gonads, leading to sex hormone secretion.

In the male, the testes enlarge and testosterone (via peripheral conversion to dihydrotestosterone) produces pubic hair and penile growth. Acne, mood swings, the breaking of the voice and attainment of an adult body odour and sweat pattern are all androgen-mediated events (in both sexes).

In the female, the breasts enlarge as oestrogen is produced from the ovary. The androgenic effects that are observed (pubic and axillary hair, acne and body odour) are secondary to increased androgen secretion from the adrenal gland – 'adrenarche'. Ultrasonography reveals ovarian enlargement, follicle production and ultimately to maturation of the uterus and endometrium, followed by menstruation – 'menarche'.

For a more detailed description of the physical changes of puberty, see Chapter 4.

Further reading

Buckler JMH (1987) *The adolescent years.* Castlemead Publications, Ware.

Tanner JM (1989) *Foetus into man,* 2nd edn. Castlemead Publications, Ware.

Ulijasek JJ, Johnston FE and Preece MA (eds) (1998) *The Cambridge encyclopaedia of growth and development.* Cambridge University Press, Cambridge.

Growth charts and how to use them

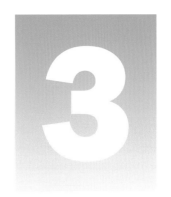

Standards and plotting

Up-to-date standards for height, weight, body mass index and head circumference are available for many populations. The current UK 1995 charts are shown below, and the data used for all of the examples in the book. These are the only charts that should be used in primary or secondary care settings.

Standards should be updated regularly (about every decade) to take into account secular changes in growth, and although ideally data on ethnic subgroups should be available for practical purposes, all children can be plotted on the same charts regardless of their racial origin.

Standards for height velocity (longitudinal data), sitting height, leg length, skinfold thickness span, etc., are based on older data (1950s to 1970s), but are still used in some specialist growth clinics. The older cross-sectional height and weight charts derived by Tanner and Whitehouse are now obsolete and should not be used.

The most commonly used charts are sex-specific and show the measured parameter on the vertical axis and age on the horizontal axis. Almost all scales are linear, except for skinfold thickness, where a vertical logarithmic axis is used because the value is not normally distributed.

Height and weight charts are 'cross-sectional' – that is, they are constructed from observations of large numbers of individuals of each sex at given ages, measured once only. The frequency distribution of height and weight is then converted into a percentile ('centile') plot, which is smoothed to produce the familiar growth curve (see Figure 3.1).

Preterm growth charts are constructed from cross-sectional birth weights and lengths of babies born before 37 weeks, so the curve derived from this data may not be appropriate for assessing postnatal weight gain.

Charts of height and weight in many of the more common named syndromic conditions are available (e.g. Down's syndrome, Turner's syndrome, Noonan's syndrome) and should be used where necessary. There are also charts of limb length, height and occipitofrontal circumference (OFC) for many of the skeletal dysplasias.

Fig 3.1
Construction of one 'age' band for a cross-sectional growth chart. Hundreds of children of the same age and sex are measured, and a frequency distribution of their height is plotted as shown. Height has a 'normal' distribution (the familiar bell-shaped curve). Centiles can be calculated and are related to SD as indicated on the lower linear scale. The centile plot is then rotated by 90 degrees, to provide one age/centile distribution for the chart. The process is repeated for further ages, and the centile points on each are joined by a smoothed line to produce the familiar growth charts.

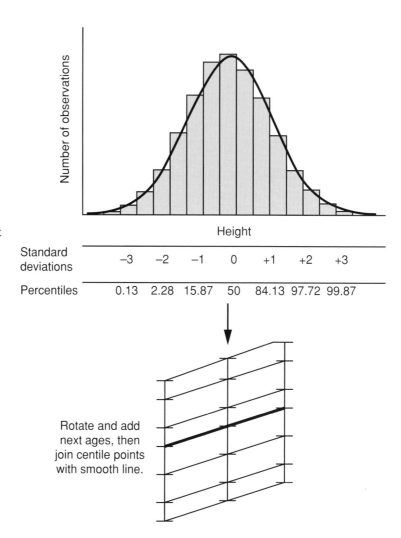

It is necessary to understand the concept of standard deviation scores in order to appreciate the detail of construction of the charts.

To allow more precise quantification of any normally distributed parameter for which standards exist, it is common to use the standard deviation score (SDS or Z-score), especially for values that lie outside the normal centile range. This technique allows comparison of the parameters for children of different age and sex.

$$Z\text{-score or SDS} = \frac{x - \bar{x}}{\text{SD}}$$

where x is the measured value, x̄ is the mean and SD is the standard deviation for a given population. For a value that is normally distributed in the population, such as height, the SDS will have a mean of 0 and an SD of 1. An SDS of −1 to +1 includes 68.26% and an SDS of −2 to +2 includes 95.44% of the population. Only 0.13% of a population will have an SDS of more or less than 3.

The currently used UK height charts (see Figure 3.2) are constructed with centile lines spaced equally approximately two-thirds of a standard deviation apart. This results in lines equivalent to the 0.4th and 99.6th (= ± 2.66 SD), 2nd and 98th (± 2.0 SD), 9th and 91st (± 1.32 SD) and 25th and 75th (± 0.66 SD) centiles below and above the mean (50th centile, 0 SD). Thus the extremes of normality for the purposes of height screening can be set at < 0.4th or > 99.6th % (i.e. only 1 in 250 healthy children will fall outside these limits).

Weight is *not* normally distributed (see Figure 3.2), as there are more heavy than light individuals, so the lines on the weight chart are not evenly spaced, but otherwise the same constraints apply.

The BMI chart (see Figure 3.3) describes the relationship of the derived ratio weight/height^2 against age, and is constructed in the same way as described above from the calculated values derived from real population observations.

All values on growth charts should be plotted as a simple dot, and other values, such as bone age (see below) should be plotted in a different colour or with a square symbol. Do not use crosses, circles or 'donuts' as symbols as they obscure data in frequent plots and are less accurate for recording measurements (see Figure 3.4)!

Pay particular attention to the horizontal scale. In premature neonates as many as 30% of measurements are wrongly plotted on the horizontal axis because of failure to calculate age accurately. In the first 2 years allow for prematurity by adjusting the plot on the X-axis. Horizontal axes may be provided as days/weeks (for premature babies to term), weeks/months (up to 2 years), months/years (up to 20 years) or as decimals of a year (see below).

In specialist clinics where frequent measurements and follow-up are likely, age is often calculated as a decimal. Birthday and current date can be looked up in a decimal age chart (see Figure 3.5) and subtracted to give the exact age at measurement.

Box 3.1 Use of decimal age (1)	
Current date	2001.46
Date of birth	1998.33
Age	3.13 years

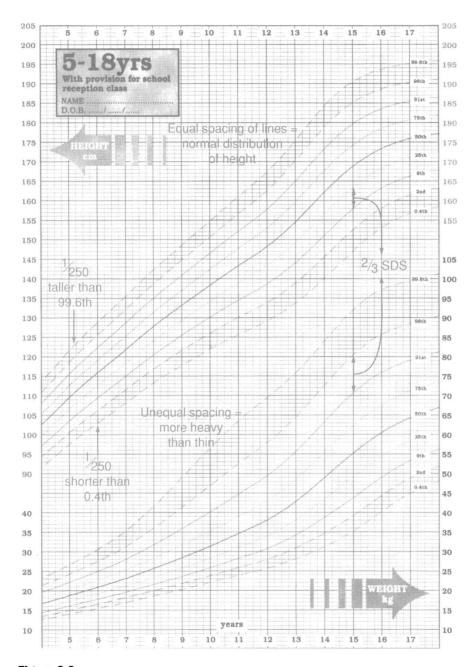

Figure 3.2
UK charts based on data collected in 1990 and published in 1995. Equal spacing of nine height centile lines 2/3 standard deviation apart. Weight is not normally distributed, as there are more heavy than light individuals in a population, so the nine centile lines are unequally spaced.

Referral guidelines

Refer a girl whose BMI falls above the 98th centile as obese. Consider referral, as overweight, a girl whose BMI falls above the 91st centile even on the basis of a single measurement. Consider for referral a girl whose BMI falls below the 2nd centile as being significantly underweight even on the basis of a single measurement. During infancy large but transient changes in centile may occur due to the shape of the charts, and these changes are normal. It should be remembered that the earlier the age of the second rise, the greater the risk of future obesity. Remember also that while BMI has a high correlation with relative fatness or leanness it is actually assessing the weight-to-height relationship: **this may give misleading results in girls who are very stocky and muscular who might appear obese on the BMI alone.**

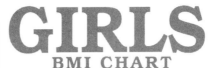

How to calculate BMI
Divide weight (kg) by square of length/height (m²) e.g. when weight = 25kg and length/height = 1.2m (120cm), BMI = 25 ÷ (1.2 x 1.2) = 17.4

Date	Age	Length/Height	Weight	BMI	Initials
: :	: :	:	:	:	:
: :	: :	:	:	:	:
: :	: :	:	:	:	:
: :	: :	:	:	:	:
: :	: :	:	:	:	:
: :	: :	:	:	:	:
: :	: :	:	:	:	:

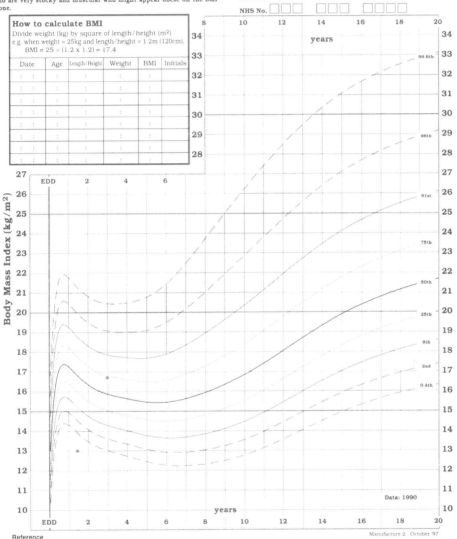

Reference
Body Mass Index reference curves for the UK, 1990 (TJ Cole, JV Freeman, MA Preece) *Arch Dis Child* 1995; **73**: 25-29
Sex differences in weight in infancy (MA Preece, JV Freeman, TJ Cole) *BMJ* 1996; **313**: 1486

Figure 3.3

BMI (and skinfold thickness) bears a non-linear relationship to age. There is rapid accumulation of fat postnatally, followed by a slimming down as a toddler becomes more physically active and picky about food. There is a 'puppy-fat' stage prior to puberty, followed by accumulation of more sexual fat during puberty, and finally a stabilisation to adult BMI values at the end of sexual development. Only in adulthood does the numerical rule of thumb 'BMI of 22 is ideal, BMI greater than 28 is overweight', familiar from cardiovascular risk charts become appropriate.

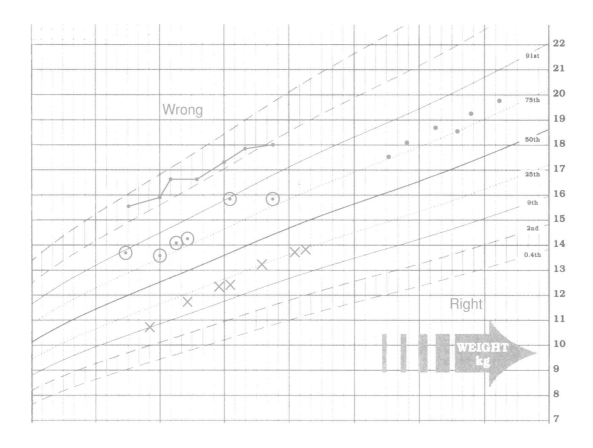

Figure 3.4
Crosses, dots with circles and lines joining points all obscure data and should not be used. A simple dot is all that is required.

Target height and OFC

Ideally, both parents should be measured directly (see Chapter 2). Remember that non-paternity may be present in 5–20% of cases!

Box 3.2   Target height

The genetic potential or mid-parental height (MPH) of a child is calculated simply by the following formulae.

Target height for boy = ([father's height + mother's height]/2) + 7 cm.
Target height for girl = ([mother's height + father's height]/2) – 7 cm.

The worked calculation is provided on the current UK charts, shown here for a female. In a male (e) would read '= (d) + 7 cm and the TCR in (g) would be ± 10 cm (see Figure 3.6).

DECIMAL YEAR CALCULATION

	1	2	3	4	5	6	7	8	9	10	11	12	13	14	15	16	17	18	19	20	21	22	23	24	25	26	27	28	29	30	31
JAN	000	003	005	008	011	014	016	019	022	025	027	030	033	036	038	041	044	047	049	052	055	058	060	063	066	068	071	074	077	079	082
FEB	085	088	090	093	096	099	101	104	107	110	112	115	118	121	123	126	129	132	134	137	140	142	145	148	151	153	156	159			
MAR	162	164	167	170	173	175	178	181	184	186	189	192	195	197	200	203	205	208	211	214	216	219	222	225	227	230	233	236	238	241	244
APR	247	249	252	255	258	260	263	266	268	271	274	277	279	282	285	288	290	293	296	299	301	304	307	310	312	315	318	321	323	326	
MAY	329	332	334	337	340	342	345	348	351	353	356	359	362	364	367	370	373	375	378	381	384	386	389	392	395	397	400	403	405	408	411
JUN	414	416	419	422	425	427	430	433	436	438	441	444	447	449	452	455	458	460	463	466	468	471	474	477	479	482	485	488	490	493	
JUL	496	499	501	504	507	510	512	515	518	521	523	526	529	532	534	537	540	542	545	548	551	553	556	559	562	564	567	570	573	575	578
AUG	581	584	586	589	592	595	597	600	603	605	608	611	614	616	619	622	625	627	630	633	636	638	641	644	647	649	652	655	658	660	663
SEPT	666	668	671	674	677	679	682	685	688	690	693	696	699	701	704	707	710	712	715	718	721	723	726	729	731	734	737	740	742	745	
OCT	748	751	753	756	759	762	764	767	770	773	775	778	781	784	786	789	792	795	797	800	803	805	808	811	814	816	819	822	825	827	830
NOV	833	836	838	841	844	847	849	852	855	858	860	863	866	868	871	874	877	879	882	885	888	890	893	896	899	901	904	907	910	912	
DEC	915	918	921	923	926	929	932	934	937	940	942	945	948	951	953	956	959	962	964	967	970	973	975	978	981	984	986	989	992	995	997

Figure 3.5
Decimal calendar from current UK charts.

ADULT HEIGHT POTENTIAL

The table and illustrations below show how the adult height potential of a girl is calculated. They show that if she follows her genetic growth pattern corrected for gender (see a-e) she should reach 164cm as an adult - her **mid-parent corrected height [MPH]**. The arrow (h) indicates that her **mid-parental centile [MPC]** is the 50th centile and her growth curve should border this centile from approximately the age of 2yrs. If it borders an adjacent centile her growth will still lie within her **target centile range [TCR]** - MPH ± 8.5cm (g): if it falls outside the TCR however she should be referred for a medical check. NB This calculation is not appropriate if either parent is not of normal stature.

Complete the Adult Height Potential Calculation Table
on Chart 4 as follows:-

(a) = father's height
(b) = mother's height
(c) = sum of (a) and (b)
(d) = (c) ÷ 2
(e) = (d) - 7cm (**MPH**)
(f) = **MPC** - nearest centile to (e)
(g) = **TCR** (mid-parental height ± 8.5cm)

Arrow (h) the mid-parental height/centile in the area above the Adult Height Calculation Table and draw a vertical line above and below it to represent the target centile range.

(a)   ....186...cm
(b)   ....156...cm
(c)   ....342..cm
(d)   ....171...cm
(e)   ...164..cm   (f) ....50th....centile
(g)   ....91st.centile — ....9th...centile

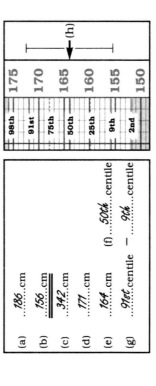

98th	175
91st	170
75th	165
50th	160 (h)
25th	160
9th	155
2nd	150

Figure 3.6

Worked calculation as shown on 1995 UK charts.

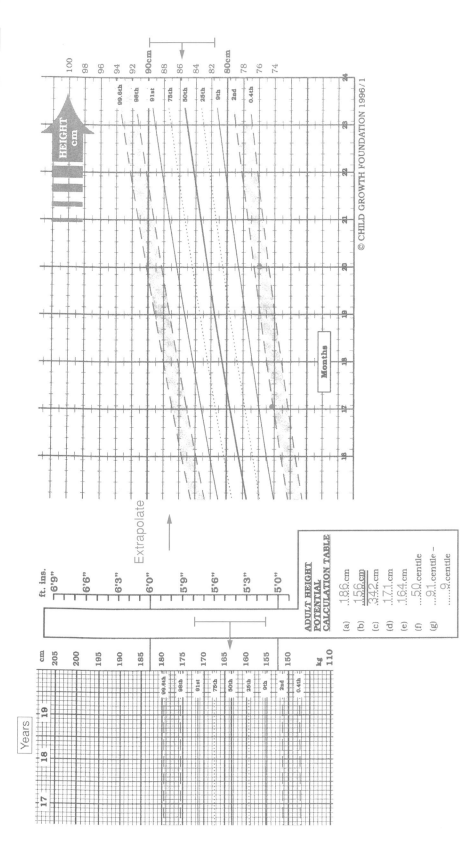

© CHILD GROWTH FOUNDATION 1996/1

HEIGHT cm

Months

Extrapolate

Years

ADULT HEIGHT POTENTIAL CALCULATION TABLE

(a) ...1.86.cm
(b) ...1.56.cm
(c) ...3.42.cm
(d) ...1.71.cm
(e) ...1.64.cm
(f) ...50.centile
(g) ...9.1.centile -
    ......9.centile

Figure 3.7

It is possible to extrapolate from the centiles at the mid-point and extremes of target range to any other chart (e.g. less than 2 years, Turner's syndrome; see later) and gain a reasonably meaningful idea of genetic potential and range for a child using genetic data that has been adjusted to that age or condition by the use of centiles. Remember that a child will not achieve his or her full genetic position until the age of 2 years, so use of this calculation during the first year is of less value unless it is weighted towards the mother's size.

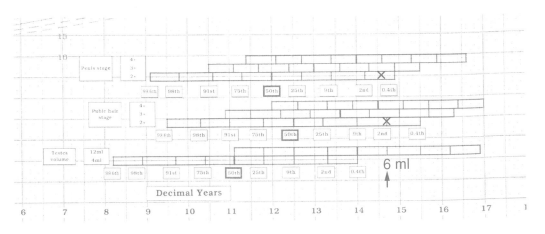

Figure 3.15
Detail from UK charts showing centiles for timing of male sexual development. The plotted example is of a boy aged 14¾ years presenting with moderately severe delay, 6 mL testes, stage 2 pubic hair and penis. He has started puberty, and so long as 'arrested' puberty is excluded by history/examination (see later), it is likely that he will start a growth spurt during the next year. Given the pubertal signs, it is probably not necessary to perform the bone age, but it would probably be delayed, being equivalent to about 12 years.

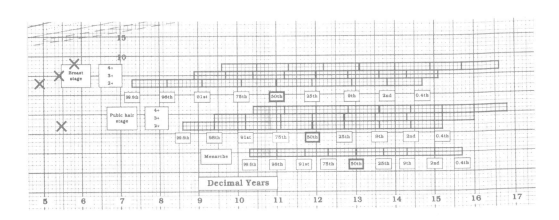

Figure 3.16
Detail from UK charts showing centiles for timing of female sexual development. The plotted example is equivalent to Figure 3.14A, showing early breast and pubic hair development (but no periods yet) in a girl with central precocious puberty.

Tempo of growth

Because of the sex-hormone-augmented growth of the back and increased secretion of growth hormone, the pubertal height spurt is dependent on the timing of gonadal hormone production. There is a variation in this timing, as for all biological parameters, such that some individuals mature earlier and some mature later than their contemporaries. An allowance is made for this variation in tempo on the height velocity chart, where early and late developers are denoted by the shaded area on each side of the artificially aligned 'peak' height velocity (see Figure 3.10). It is perfectly possible for a first-year senior-school class of girls to contain an immature female and a fully menstruating female, as well as the majority in mid-puberty, and for a class of 14-year-old boys to include both immature and shaving individuals. This also means that some children will have 'shot-up' with an early spurt and will be 20–30 cm taller than their late-developing friends, who will eventually catch up (see Figure 3.17). Delayed puberty is one of the commonest reasons for concern, and will be discussed separately in Chapter 4.

There is a secular trend towards earlier puberty, especially in societies such as ours where relative over-nutrition is common.

What information can you obtain from a growth chart?

It is no exaggeration to say that 90% of the diagnosis of a growth problem can come from a carefully taken history and reliable data plotted on the appropriate charts.

First, the height and weight of a child can be seen in comparison with those for the UK population of the same age and sex. They may be relatively short or tall, or within the normal range (see Figure 3.18).

Secondly, what is the relationship of their weight to their height (see Figure 3.19)? Are they relatively heavy and short, tall and thin, or tall and heavy? All of these patterns may increase the likelihood of pathology, as we shall see in the following chapters.

If a bone age has been obtained, or sexual maturation is occurring, one can estimate their remaining growth and hence their height potential (see Figure 3.20).

Then it needs to be established whether in comparison to their parent(s) and sibling(s) they are short or tall. Are they likely to achieve their predicted adult height, given their degree of bony or sexual maturation (see Figure 3.21)?

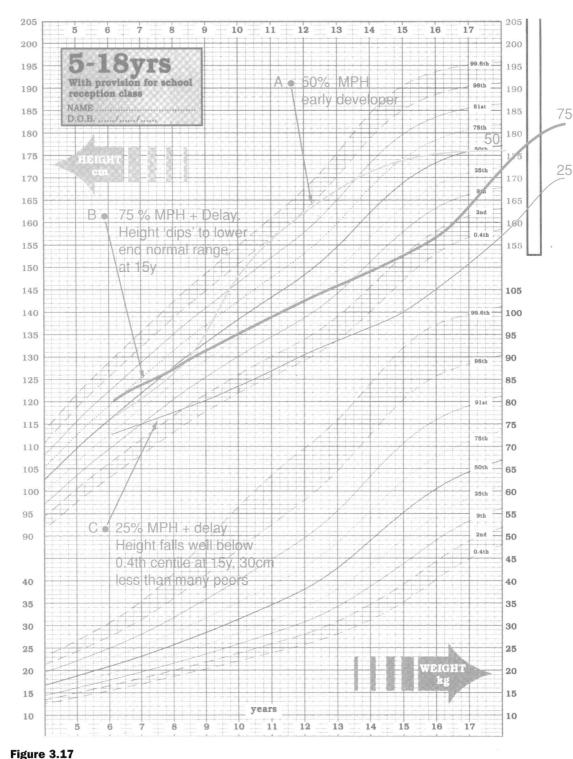

Figure 3.17

Comparison of (A) 50th centile early developer with (B) 75th centile late developer and (C) 25th centile late developer. Although the boys all reach their predicted height, the 25th centile late developer in particular is disadvantaged compared with his normally developing peers.

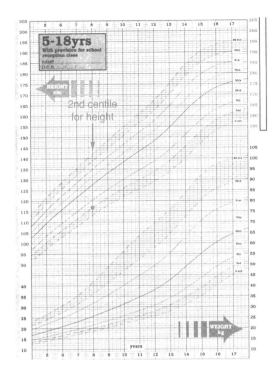

Figure 3.18

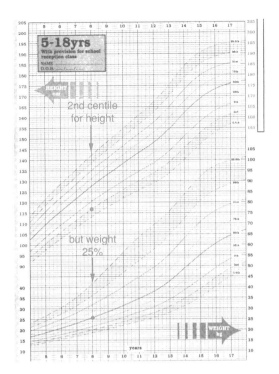

Figure 3.19

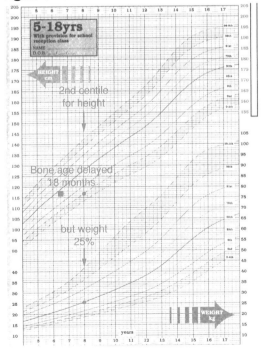

Figure 3.20

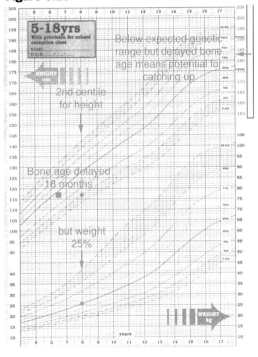

Figure 3.21

All of this information may be obtained from a single visit

If measured sequentially, then the height and weight velocity can be estimated, or any change in the relationship between these values and the starting centile noted. For a short child, a normal height velocity or catch-up with a high height velocity is very reassuring, but a low height velocity indicates the need for further investigation. Likewise, for a tall child a normal height velocity excludes progressive acquired causes of pathological tall stature that would cause an accelerating height velocity.

If sitting height has been measured and leg length calculated, is there any short-limbed disproportion that might indicate a skeletal dysplasia or a short back as may be seen in scoliosis and some storage and connective tissue disorders (see Chapter 4)? Are the legs just relatively long in comparison to the back? (This is commonly seen in delayed puberty, because GH secretion is normal, so the long bones of the leg have continued to grow, but the back has stayed relatively short because of the lack of sex steroids) (see Figure 3.22d).

At follow-up (see Figure 3.23) the three possibilities are catch-up (which is reassuring), maintenance of centile position (which implies a normal height velocity, and in the absence of any new symptoms or concerns should be treated expectantly) or poor growth (which is pathological and needs urgent investigation even in the absence of symptoms) (see Chapter 4).

Community screening for short and tall stature

There has been much emotive debate about the routine screening of length/height and growth rates in the general population. After reading this manual I hope the reader will be persuaded that opportunistic measurement of height should form part of the routine examination of any child presenting for medical attention. However, there is a lack of evidence that measurement of healthy children, in the absence of parental concern, is of any benefit to the individual, or that serial estimation of the growth rate increases the detection of treatable causes of growth failure.

Information about the public health and social circumstances of a *population*, and their secular trends, can certainly be of great benefit to society, but very few asymptomatic individuals with treatable forms of growth failure will be detected by mass screening.

Because of the inaccuracies inherent in measurement, serial height estimations magnify error and render interpretation of height velocity outside specialist units fraught with danger. Conversely, it is clear that if

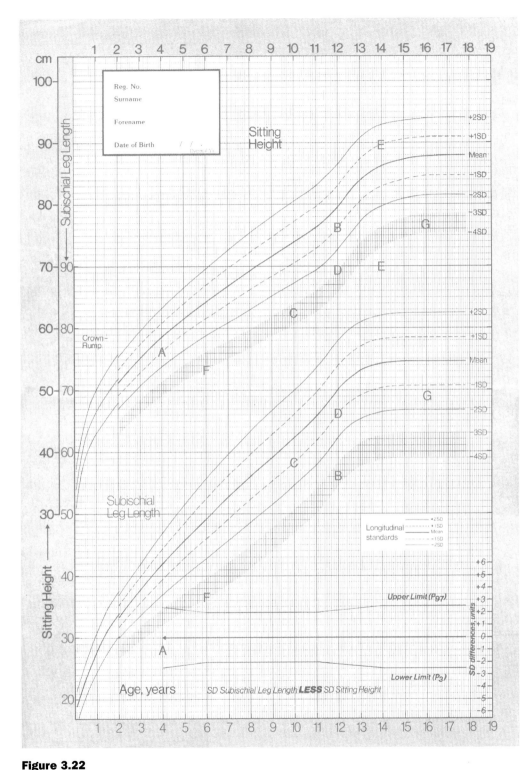

Figure 3.22
(A) Achondroplasia. (B) Hypochondroplasia. (C) Scoliosis or storage disorder. (D) Delayed puberty/hypogonadism. (E) Marfan's syndrome. (F) Short, proportionate child (e.g. Turner's syndrome). (G) Juvenile case of Hunter's syndrome.

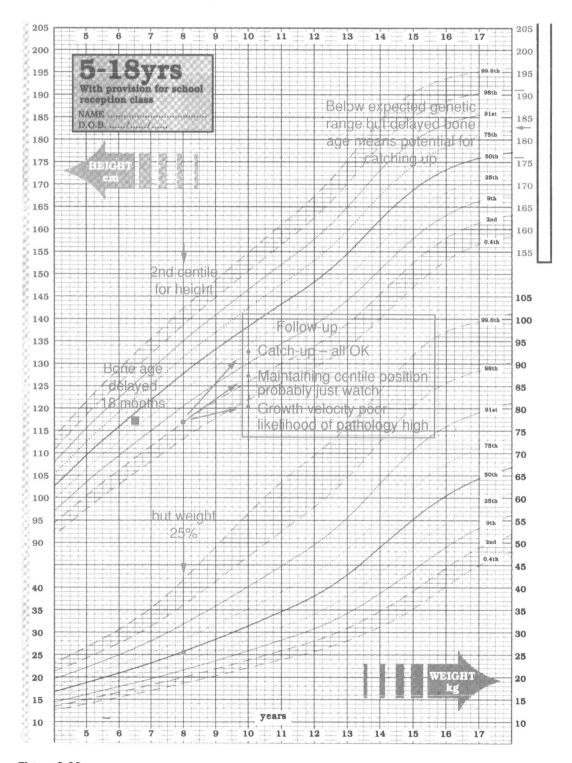

Figure 3.23

Table 3.1

Screening for short stature

Condition	Approximate frequency	Age and height at diagnosis	Benefits of early diagnosis	Conclusion
Isolated growth hormone deficiency (GHD) or multiple pituitary hormone deficiency (MPHD)	1:3500 to 1:2000, including mild/borderline cases. Incidence declining in recent years (possibly due to better obstetric care)	Isolated GHD presents at mean age 5.5 (1.2) years with height SDS of –3 (0.2) (MPHD presents at age 2.8 (0.6) years with height SDS of –4 (0.2). Around 88% of GHD cases present with growth failure prior to the age of 5 years	GH therapy necessary to achieve optimal final height. Delayed treatment may result in reduced final height	Screening at school entry to identify cases that do not present earlier might identify over 60% of available cases. Additional yield of further measurements is probably small
Turner's syndrome	1:2000 female births	Significant number (40%?) of cases found at or before birth. Growth rate fairly normal in first 4 years of life. The 0.4th centile (–2.66 SD) cut-off identifies 56% of cases at age 5 years. Yield increases to 80% if parental heights are taken into account. Girls with the disorder are on average 18–22 cm below MPH at final height	Early treatment may improve final height. Psychological benefits possibly more important	Measuring at age 5 years could detect half to two-thirds of cases that are not found earlier. Further height measures are unlikely to detect many more cases before puberty
Acquired hypothyroidism	1:6000 or less	Few data are available. Mean height at diagnosis –1.18 SD; mean weight –0.12 SD. Only 3 in 10 cases more than –2 SD (below 2nd centile), and only 1 in 10 more than –2.66 SD (< 0.4th centile)	Eminently treatable condition, but catch-up growth is often unsatisfactory, even once diagnosed (see Chapter 4). Children below 0.4th centile (more than –2.66 SD) merit exclusion of hypothyroidism, but this does not justify screening or growth monitoring	It is unlikely that height alone would identify such cases, but no data are available

Table 3.1 continued

Condition	Approximate frequency	Age and height at diagnosis	Benefits of early diagnosis	Conclusion
Inflammatory bowel disease	4:100 000 children under 16 years of age per year	Crohn's disease may present with poor growth: mean height at presentation −1.11 (±1.28) SD and 21% more than −1.88 SD (< 3rd centile). Delay in diagnosis averages 7 months; 13% of cases have height more than −2.0 SDS	Early treatment is desirable, but there is no evidence that a few months' delay alters the outcome	Growth failure in the absence of other symptoms is a very uncommon situation. Growth monitoring is not justified on this basis
Coeliac disease	1:2000, but recent data suggest that it may be more common than this	Height at diagnosis −1.8 SD; none more than −3 SD. Another study found 30% < −2 SD. One series had severe growth retardation	Asymptomatic short stature is unusual. Early treatment is desirable but catch-up growth is observed on a gluten-free diet	Most cases are symptomatic. Growth monitoring is not justified for detection of rare cases with isolated short stature
Chronic renal disease	1:50 000?	Might present as growth impairment	Early diagnosis is important to reduce compli-cations. Most cases are symptomatic	Growth monitoring is not justified for detection of rare cases with isolated short stature
Noonan's syndrome	1:2000	Mean height and final height −2 SD. Other features may prompt investigation	Early diagnosis might prevent much parental distress. Associated heart and clotting abnormalities may be detected	Most cases are symptomatic. Growth monitoring is not justified for detection of rare cases with isolated short stature
Achondroplasia, other skeletal dysplasias and bone disorders	1:15 000– 1:77 000	Most present due to other features. There are no data on how many mild cases (hypo-chondroplasia) present in childhood	Early diagnosis might prevent much parental distress. Can be entered into surgical leg-lengthening programme	Most cases are symptomatic. Growth monitoring is not justified for detection of rare cases with isolated short stature

Adapted from DMB Hall, personal communication, with permission.

Table 3.2
Screening for tall stature

Condition	Approximate frequency	Age and height at diagnosis	Benefits of early diagnosis	Conclusion
Marfan's syndrome	1:10 000	32 out of 40 children ≥ +1.88 SD. Most present with tall stature plus other classic musculoskeletal features	Early intervention may extend life expectancy (beta-blockade to prevent dilatation of aorta)	Awareness of tall stature and musculoskeletal features could facilitate early recognition. A single height measure would suffice
Klinefelter's syndrome, XXY	1.3:1000 male births	Tall, but there are insufficient data to estimate how many more than + 2 SD. Arm span exceeds height. Increased velocity between 5 and 8 years of age due to increased leg growth	Early diagnosis might prevent much distress. Two-thirds of cases remain undiagnosed	Growth monitoring is not justified for identifying XXY
XYY	1:1000 male births	Increased velocity and final height, but no detailed data are available	85% of cases remain undiag-nosed. Value of early diagnosis is uncertain	Growth monitoring is not justified for identifying XYY
Thyrotoxicosis	Incidence about 1:100 000 children	Increased height velocity; usually other features	Insufficient evidence is available	Too rare to merit growth monitoring
Sotos' syndrome	Rare	Height usually more than + 2 SD in childhood, but final height is not hugely increased	May allow early planning of educational needs	Usually diagnosed by other features (e.g. large head)
Pituitary gigantism	Very rare	Likely to be very tall: other features such as field defects also present	Beneficial	Too rare to merit growth monitoring

Adapted from DMB Hall, personal communication, with permission.

opportunistic measurements show a falling off of height centile position, or excessively rapid growth, then a cause should be sought. Why should there be this apparent discrepancy?

A screening procedure should only be undertaken if the condition is common and treatable and if no harm befalls those who are falsely detected as positive cases (among many other criteria). However, most treatable causes of growth failure or excess growth *that do not present with overt symptomatology* are rare, and are listed in Tables 3.1 and 3.2 with approximate incidence figures.

Of these conditions only about 50% of Turner's syndrome girls will fall below the 0.4th centile at 5 years, although up to 40% will have been detected earlier with heart abnormalities or dysmorphic features (see later), so only about one girl with Turner's syndrome/10 000 subjects screened will be detected (see Figure 3.24).

A better case can be made for screening for GHD, as more than two-thirds of cases of idiopathic GHD will show growth failure by 5 years of age

Figure 3.24
Turner's syndrome: 3–97% lines superimposed on UK 1995 female centile chart. Around 50% of girls will be identified as 'short – less than 0.4%' at 5 years of age. If parental size is taken into account, then the majority of cases will be detected. Reproduced from DMB Hall with permission.

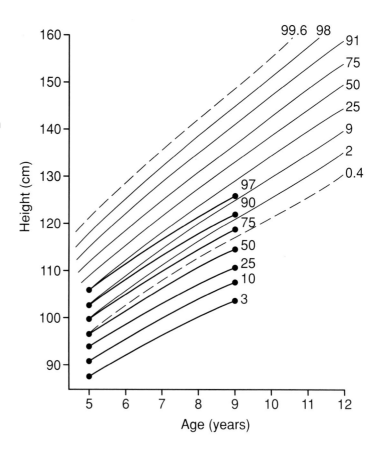

and so be detected by a single measurement. Therefore perhaps 1 in 4000–5000 cases screened will be found. However, late-onset coeliac disease and hypothyroidism, which are very treatable, rarely cause extreme growth failure and will be missed, especially as their onset may occur after 5 years of age.

Thus the current recommendation is that all children should be measured once, at school entry, with well-maintained equipment used by well-trained individuals. Those children whose height falls below the 0.4th centile should be referred for assessment. Guidelines for referral or follow-up of tall, fat or thin individuals are less clear-cut.

Further reading

Hall DMB (2001) *Health for all children*, 4th edn. Oxford University Press, Oxford.

Schilig S and Hulse A (2000). *Growth assessment in the community*, 3rd edn. Child Growth Foundation, London.

Wales JKH, Wit JM and Rogol AD (1996) *A color atlas of pediatric endocrinology and growth*. Mosby-Wolfe, London.

Short stature

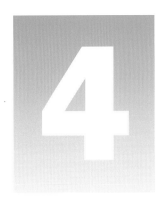

History of the child with short stature (including assessment of sexual maturity)

All diagnosis should begin with a comprehensive history and examination.

The presenting complaint as perceived by the parents should be addressed first. As always, parental concerns are dismissed at your peril. If they are old enough, ask the patient whether *they* have any concerns, too, or if this is only a problem to other family members or health professionals.

Important points include the following:

- Details of the pregnancy – ill health or drug administration, gestational age, mode of delivery, any requirement for neonatal special care, birth weight, birth length and head circumference from parent-held or hospital records;
- growth rate in terms of height – as recorded in past medical records or by parents; is the child growing out of their clothes and shoes before they wear out?
- growth rate in terms of weight – is there weight loss or a steady gain in weight despite poor height growth?
- family tree – parental heights (preferably measured directly) – beware of dominantly inherited disorders such as hypochondroplasia; parental build, age of menarche, sexual maturation of father in relation to his peers (e.g. voice breaking or shaving), marked short stature, consanguinity (this leads to an increased risk of autosomal-recessive disorders);
- other ill health – especially autoimmune problems (rheumatoid arthritis, pernicious anaemia, alopecia, vitiligo) or 'glands'; specifically enquire about thyroid disorders and insulin- or non-insulin-dependent diabetes mellitus;
- social details – important for assessment of failure to thrive and later compliance with treatment;
- medication – ask about *any* regular treatment (including topical and inhaled preparations);

Figure 4.1
Example of an 'informative' family tree, showing autoimmune disease on the mother's side, average parental height and no history of major delay in puberty. This illustrative case may have hypothyroidism.

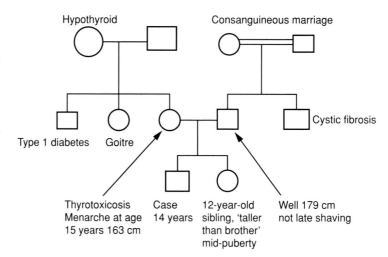

- specific questions – headache and visual disturbance (as may be found in craniopharyngioma);
- past medical events – including even what might be perceived as minor surgical procedures, such as hernia repair or orchidopexy (there may be unrecognized testicular damage, or the hernia may be part of a syndromic association);
- dietary history – including early milk feeding, age of weaning and any specific exclusions from the diet (this is particularly true if you are assessing obesity or failure to thrive, when a question such as, 'What did you give him to eat yesterday?' followed by a specific question about each item at each meal may provide a lot of information) (see Chapters 8 and 9);
- developmental or educational level;
- pubertal timing and progression in child (if present);
- participation in sport;
- bullying;
- career plans – for example, if the child wants to be a jockey or a basketball player, that may be very important and some careers have exclusions on grounds of short stature or ill health;
- system review – to exclude other pathology.

Examination of the child with short stature (including assessment of sexual maturity)

Observe the child's activity, demeanour and interaction with their parents or carers.

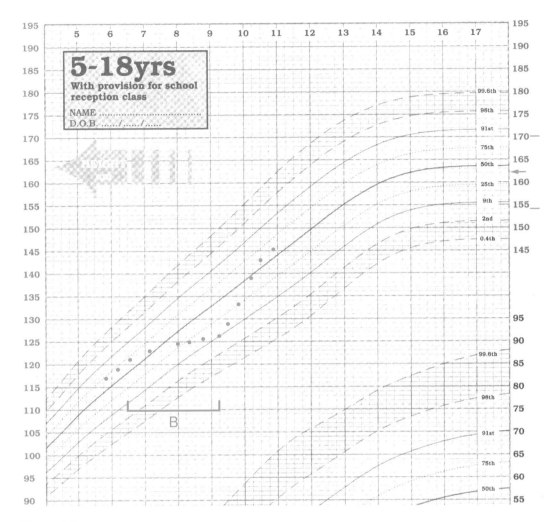

Figure 4.2
Growth failure consequent upon inhaled beclomethasone (B), 100 μg twice a day. There is recovery of growth on switching to a non-steroidal preventer.

*Note: in the following, items marked * are found in several dysmorphic syndromes associated with short stature.*

HANDS (FEET) AND ARMS (LEGS)

- Abnormal dermatoglyphics*.
- Loose joints and hypermobility of the wrists and fingers – seen in some of the collagen disorders.

- Joint stiffness – may be seen in longstanding diabetes mellitus and some of the storage disorders.
- Joint contractures – may be restricted to one group of joints (various syndromes* and storage disorders) or generalized*.
- Generally short fingers (brachydactyly) – various syndromes*.
- Only one or two short metacarpals – Turner's syndrome or (more markedly) pseudohypoparathyroidism.
- Fusion (syndactyly) – various syndromes*.
- Duplication with or without fusion (polydactyly or polysyndactyly) – various syndromes*.
- All of the fingers bent (camptodactyly) – various syndromes*.
- Bent fifth finger (clinodactyly) – various syndromes*.
- Trident hand – skeletal dysplasias.
- Thumb abnormal (broad, triphalangeal or low set) – various syndromes*.
- Clubbing – chronic cyanotic heart disease; chronic purulent respiratory disorders; inflammatory bowel disease; dominant in some families with normal stature.
- One or all nails may be hypoplastic – (syndromes characterized by early lymphoedema, such as Turner's syndrome, cause puffy feet/hands *in utero* and hence small nails).
- Palms:
  yellowish discoloration – hypothyroidism;
  redness – chronic liver disorders.
- Wrist expanded – rickets.
- Limited rotation of forearm – some skeletal dysplasias.
- Radial aplasia or hypoplasia – associated with congenital heart defects, renal or haematological abnormalities*.
- Increased carrying angle – seen in 50% of Turner's syndrome cases (and may be present in other syndromes*).

NECK

- Loose skin – Down's, Turner's and other chromosomal syndromes*, again those associated with *in-utero* lymphoedema).
- Webbing – 70% of cases of Turner's syndrome (also seen in many other dysmorphic syndromes*).
- Low posterior hair line – many syndromes*.
- Thyroid, goitre – *can be best palpated while standing behind the sitting patient, or with the patient lying with the head falling backwards slightly over the edge of the couch. Measure width and height of each lobe, listen for a bruit, feel for asymmetry (which may indicate a tumour) and feel for lymphadenopathy.*

FACE AND SKULL

- Abnormal shape* – craniosynostosis* or postural flattening.

Eyes
- Hypertelorism, epicanthic folds, ptosis – various syndromes*.

Mouth and palate
Submucous cleft palate may only be revealed by palpation.
Note: any abnormalities of the mid-line are especially significant as they may indicate an associated abnormality of the pituitary gland.

- High arched palate – Turner's, Noonan's and some other dysmorphic syndromes*.
- Smooth tongue – iron deficiency and pernicious anaemia.
- Aberrant lingual thyroid tissue may be visible.
- Swollen and 'fish-like' lips – Crohn's disease.
- Oral candidiasis – type 1 diabetes mellitus, immunodeficiency associated with hypoparathyroidism (DiGeorge's syndrome), autoimmune polyglandular type I or 'HAM' syndrome of hypoparathyroidism, adrenal failure and moniliasis.
- Teeth:
  soft and carious – disorders affecting collagen, fibrin and calcium metabolism;
  peg-like – ectodermal dysplasia;
  other abnormal shape – various syndromes*;
  stained or rotted – drugs, sugar content of diet/drugs and bilirubin;
  single central incisor – congenital growth hormone deficiency.

Note: an assessment of the presence and number of the primary dentition and the appearance of the secondary teeth can give clues to skeletal age and physiological maturity. Delayed eruption of the teeth is seen in any disorder that delays physical maturation (especially chronic disease, hypothyroidism and hypopituitarism), in cleido-cranial dysostosis and in some other dysmorphic syndromes associated with short stature.

- Ears low-set with or without rotation, or folded in an abnormal manner – various syndromes*.
- Head hair:
  abnormally sparse or curled – various syndromes*;
  abnormal patterns of whorl formation – various syndromes*;
  alopecia – autoimmune disease;
  temporal hair loss – hypothyroidism.

- Pale conjunctivae – anaemia.
- Eyelashes (sparsity, duplication or luxuriance) – various syndromes*.

CHEST/CARDIOVASCULAR SYSTEM

- Exclude cystic fibrosis and other severe chronic disorders.
- Exclude major heart abnormality.
- Hypertension (generalized) – CNS tumours, neurofibromatosis, phaeo-chromocytoma (although blood pressure rise may be paroxysmal) and other adrenal disorders.
  Hypertension in right arm only and absent femorals – coarctation of the aorta, present in 40% of girls with Turner's syndrome.
- Chest shape:
  pectus excavatum or pectus carinatum – various syndromes*;
  rachitic rosary – rickets.
- Scoliosis or kyphoscoliosis – storage disorders, syndromic malformations and disorders of bone and collagen (*any loss of height can be quantified by measurement of sitting height*) (see Chapter 2).

ABDOMEN

- Abdominal organomegaly – storage disorders, thalassaemia.
- Anus:
  damaged – sexual abuse;
  tags and fissures – chronic inflammatory bowel disease.
- Herniae (or the scars of their repair early in life) – various syndromes*.

CENTRAL NERVOUS SYSTEM

- Exclude major neurological abnormality.
- Tendon reflexes, delayed relaxation – hypothyroidism.
- Optic discs:
  papilloedema – secondary to raised intracranial pressure (RICP);
  pallor and optic atrophy – local tumour or chronic RICP, or found in the DIDMOAD syndrome of **D**iabetes **I**nsipidus, **D**iabetes **M**ellitus, **O**ptic **A**trophy and **D**eafness.
- Bitemporal restriction of visual fields – craniopharyngioma.
- Retina:
  dysplastic with small optic nerve heads – septo-optic dysplasia associated with pituitary hormone deficiencies and/or mid-line brain abnormalities;
  retinitis pigmentosa – various syndromes*, storage deposits (retina or lens).
- Blue coloration of cornea – disorders of collagen metabolism.

GENERAL APPEARANCE

- Obesity – many endocrine disorders, some syndromes*, peculiar dimpled appearance in hypopituitarism.
- Body asymmetry – Russell–Silver dwarfism.
- Hemihypertrophy – increased risk of Wilms tumour.

Skin

- Neuromas or a large number (> 6) of *café-au-lait* spots – neurofibromatosis.
- Pigmentation increased (generalized or localized to scar tissue) – Addison's disease.
- Acanthosis nigricans (velvety, coal black discoloration of the axillae or neck) – insulin resistance and obesity.
- Vitiligo – commonly isolated, but may be associated with autoimmune disease.
- Bruising and skin fragility – Ehlers–Danlos syndrome (also skin laxity), Cushing's syndrome.
- Hirsutism – Cushing's syndrome and other adrenal disorders.
- Acne – Cushing's syndrome and other adrenal disorders.
- Lanugo hair – anorexia nervosa.
- Striae – Cushing's syndrome.
- Dry skin – atopic disorders, ectodermal dysplasia.
- Atrophic – various syndromes*.
- Necrobiosis lipoidica – diabetes mellitus.
- Granuloma annulare – diabetes mellitus.

PARENTS

- Many skeletal dysplasias and some dysmorphic syndromes* are dominantly inherited, and may be more obvious in later life.
- Hypo- or hyperthyroidism/goitre.
- Mild undiagnosed metabolic disorder (i.e. phenylketonuria or myotonic dystrophy) can severely affect the infant.
- Alcoholism may produce fetal alcohol syndrome.

Staging sexual development

BREAST

- Tissue and pectoralis major muscle may be absent (or destroyed by infection/surgery) – various syndromes*.
- Gynaecomastia – Klinefelter's syndrome, obesity, hyperthyroidism, tumours, hypogonadism, other syndromes*.
- Accessory nipples are common.

GENITALIA

- Shawl scrotum – various syndromes*.
- Cryptorchidism – various syndromes* (and hypogonadism).
- Hypospadias – various syndromes*.
- Imperforate hymen.

Table 4.1 Stages of sexual development in boys

	Testicular volume (mL)	Penis	Pubic hair	Comment
1	2–3	Infantile	None	Small, < 2 mL firm testes may be damaged
2	3.5–6	Lengthens	Wisps, mid-line	About 25–30 cm height gain remains
3	8–10	Broadens	Darker	Peak of growth rate
4	12–15	Not quite adult	Not quite adult	
5	20–25	Adult, with glans separate from shaft	Adult 'V'-shape	Pubic hair may later extend to thighs, and to umbilicus. Growth ceases

Table 4.2 Stages of sexual development in girls

	Menarche	Breast	Pubic hair	Comment
1	–	Infantile	None	
2	–	Breast bud felt	Wisps, mid-line	Rapid growth starts, about 20–25 cm growth remains
3	–	Breast mound visible	Darker	Peak of growth rate
4	–	Areola separate from nipple	Not quite adult	
5	+	Adult	Adult 'V'-shape	Pubic hair may later extend to thighs. Growth ceases

In all patients presenting with any growth problem a full assessment of physical maturity is *mandatory*. It is usual to stage the appearance of the pubic hair, penis and testicular volume in males, and the appearance of the breast, pubic hair and the onset of menstruation in females. Details of this staging are given in Tables 4.1 and 4.2.

Other secondary sexual characteristics should be noted, such as moodiness, acne, axillary hair, vaginal discharge and an adult body odour. Any discrepancy between the stages of sexual development in an individual are of particular importance (see Figure 4.3).

Note: puberty may start but, in the face of severe ill health, weight loss or endocrinopathy, stop again. This is known as 'arrested puberty'. Thus, as well as assessing pubertal stage, it is important to ask about the timing of the first events and examine the 'quality' of sexual development. For instance, if the testes or breasts are soft, this may indicate an interruption of testosterone/oestrogen synthesis.

Causes of short stature

Delayed puberty is by far the commonest cause for concern and referral, and is dealt with in Chapter 5.

Idiopathic short stature is defined by the absence of abnormalities in the history and physical examination. More specifically, birth weight and length are normal (as well as body proportions), there is no chronic ill health, no severe psychosocial disturbance, and a normal food intake. Idiopathic short stature is usually familial, and is characterized by the following:

- short parents;
- short stature during childhood and a reduced final height within the target range defined by parental size;
- a normal height velocity (often varying around the 25th centile – see above);
- a normal age of onset of puberty;
- bone age consistent with chronological age (within ± 2 SD).

In these cases, if the growth velocity is normal there is no need to exclude growth hormone deficiency or other pathologies by formal testing. If the growth curve deviates from the centiles, then a GH provocation test together with the screening tests described below may be indicated.

A combination of constitutional delay and genetic short stature is not uncommon. If it is combined with delayed puberty (see Chapter 5), the deficit of height compared to the peer group may be severe in early teenage

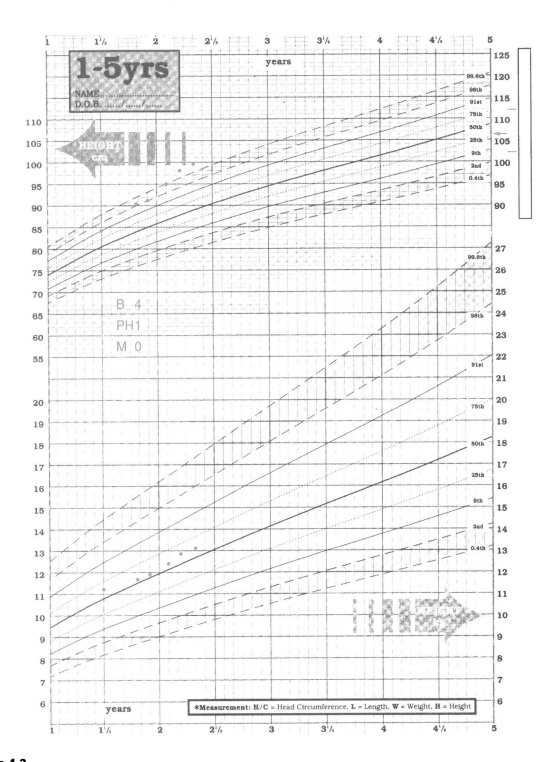

(a)

Figure 4.3

(a) Precocious breast development with no pubic hair or menses, accompanying vaginal discharge and maturation of vulval epithelium, secondary to oestrogen-secreting ovarian tumour. (b) 'Infantile hercules' with muscular body, adult body odour, acne and greasy hair. Stage 3 pubic hair, penis almost adult, but small, firm testes indicating non-gonadal source of testosterone – non-salt-wasting congenital adrenal hyperplasia.

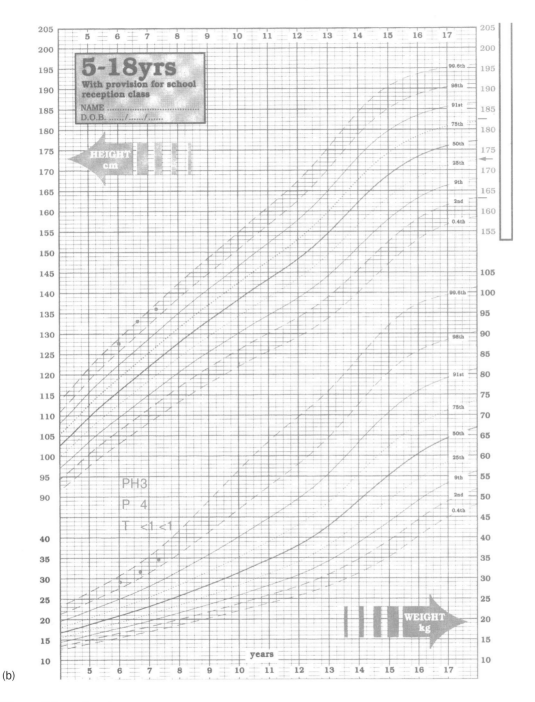

Figure 4.3 continued

Figure 4.4

Induction of pubertal growth spurt in male with delayed puberty by a 3-month course of injectable testosterone esters (T).

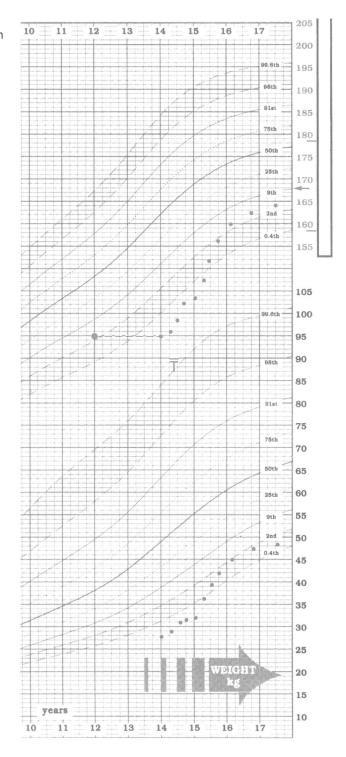

years and warrant treatment as described above, although the final height will not be influenced (see Figures 3.17 and 4.4).

The following algorithm was designed by Professor Charles Brook and has been modified by the author, with permission. The figures below are the approximate incidences of the disorders expressed as the number of years in a patient practice population of 5000 before a case would be seen by a primary care physician (see Figure 4.5).

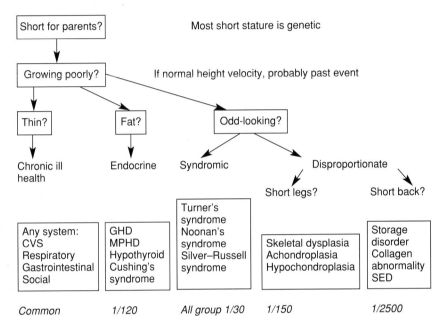

Figure 4.5
Algorithm for diagnosis of short stature. GHD, growth hormone deficiency; CVS, cardiovascular system; MPHD, multiple pituitary hormone deficiency; SED, spondyloepiphyseal dysplasia (and other dysplasias with spinal involvement).

The short and thin child

Chronic severe disorders in any system, including cardiac, lung, liver, intestinal, renal, haematological, metabolic, CNS and generalized inflammatory disease, will produce short stature and a poor growth rate while the disease process is active. Although growth hormone levels may be normal, or indeed raised, there is poor bioavailability in the presence of inflammatory cytokines, reduced oxygen availability and poor nutrition.

For example, poorly controlled diabetes may produce prepubertal short stature, wasting and delayed puberty (rarely this can occur together with hepatic dysfunction – the Mauriac syndrome).

Thinness may be even more pronounced than the short stature or poor growth rate. This may be documented as a weight centile below the height centile or a reduced BMI and low skinfold thickness (see Figure 4.6).

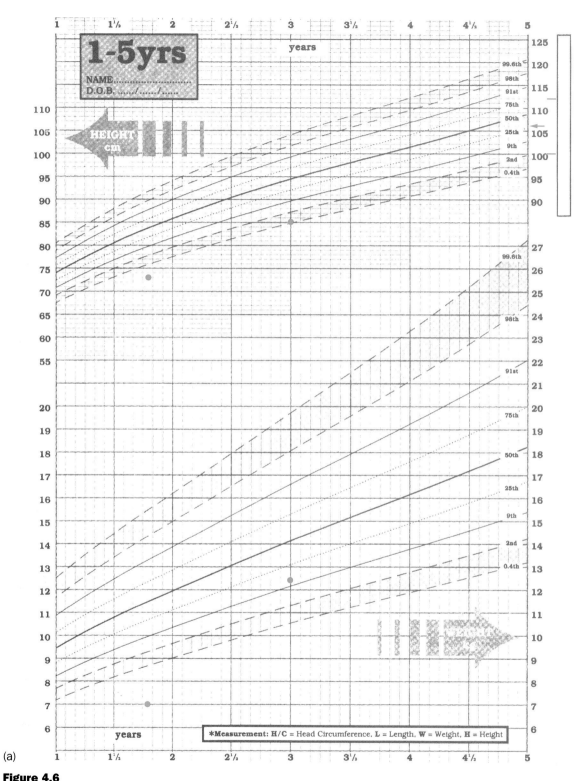

(a)

Figure 4.6

Coeliac disease at presentation and response to 1 year of exclusion diet. (a) Although this child is short for her target range, she is also thin as shown by her weight, but more obviously by (b) her BMI and (c) skinfolds.

Referral guidelines

Refer a girl whose BMI falls above the 98th centile as obese. Consider referral, as overweight, a girl whose BMI falls above the 91st centile even on the basis of a single measurement. Consider for referral a girl whose BMI falls below the 2nd centile as being significantly underweight even on the basis of a single measurement. During infancy large but transient changes in centile may occur due to the shape of the charts, and these changes are normal. It should be remembered that the earlier the age of the second rise, the greater the risk of future obesity. Remember also that while BMI has a high correlation with relative fatness or leanness it is actually assessing the weight-to-height relationship: **this may give misleading results in girls who are very stocky and muscular who might appear obese on the BMI alone.**

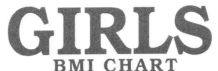

How to calculate BMI

Divide weight (kg) by square of length/height (m²)
e.g. when weight = 25kg and length/height = 1.2m (120cm),
BMI = 25 ÷ (1.2 x 1.2) = 17.4

Date		Age	Length/Height	Weight	BMI	Initials
:	:	:	:	:	:	
:	:	:	:	:	:	
:	:	:	:	:	:	
:	:	:	:	:	:	
:	:	:	:	:	:	
:	:	:	:	:	:	
:	:	:	:	:	:	
:	:	:	:	:	:	

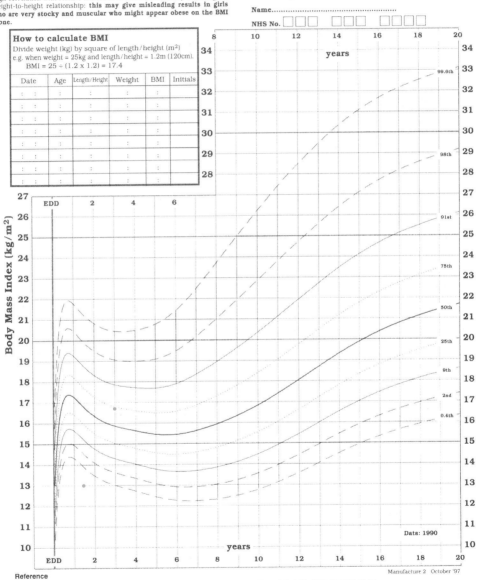

Reference
Body Mass Index reference curves for the UK, 1990 (TJ Cole, JV Freeman, MA Preece) *Arch Dis Child* 1995; **73**: 25-29
Sex differences in weight in infancy (MA Preece, JV Freeman, TJ Cole) *BMJ* 1996; **313**: 1486

(b)

Figure 4.6 continued

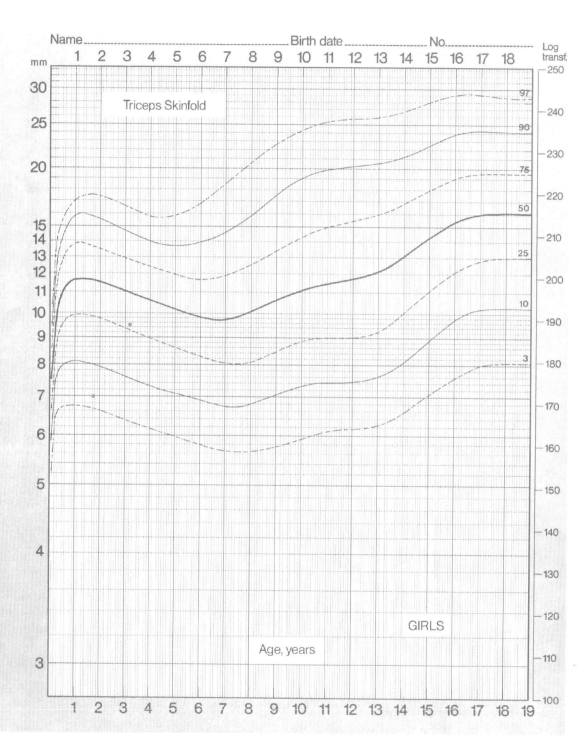

(c)

Figure 4.6 continued

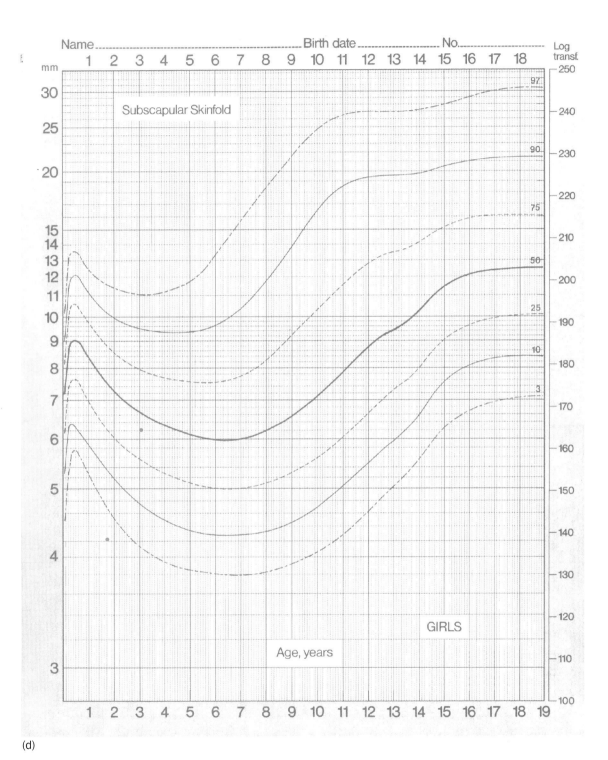

(d)

Figure 4.6 continued

Often the diagnosis will have been made before the short stature is noted. However, even in the asymptomatic child it is important to rule out hidden organic pathology.

The possibly clinically 'silent' disorders that it is most important to exclude are the following:

- renal failure, anaemia;
- infections (HIV, tuberculosis);
- inflammatory bowel diseases (e.g. Crohn's disease);
- gluten enteropathy (coeliac disease).

Psychosocial short stature (also called emotional deprivation or psycho-social dwarfism) is caused by an extremely poor emotional environment. Although there is usually relative thinness, this is not always the case, as comfort eating may occur and there can be considerable diagnostic confusion between deprivation dwarfism and GHD. Rapid catch-up growth is seen after a change of caregiver or on hospitalization (see Figure 4.7).

There is commonly a preservation of more infantile body proportions than may be expected from the age of the child. More minor degrees of short stature and thinness are a consequence of more minor deprivation and poor nutrition, which may contribute to the well-known social class gradient in height.

About 70–80% of children with intrauterine growth retardation or small-ness for dates (a birth weight less than the 2nd percentile for gestational age) reach a height and weight in the normal centiles within the first 1–2 years of postnatal life. However, 20–30% remain small, and this is an important cause of reduced stature in the adult population. The children are often thin. Asymmetrical IUGR with low birth weight but normal length is often caused by events late in pregnancy, and it usually has a good outcome. Symmetrical smallness (low weight and length) is less likely to recover, and often suggests more severe, earlier or inherent problems in the fetus or placenta, such as the following:

- genetic or metabolic disorders, e.g. chromosomal abnormalities and syndromes as described below, including Silver–Russell syndrome;
- damage *in utero* by environmental agents (infections, drugs, alcohol, maternal phenylketonuria).

Box 4.1 Silver–Russell syndrome

Prenatal growth retardation
Sparing of the head – small triangular face, thin, down-turned lips, micrognathia
Asymmetry of the limbs, clinodactyly

TREATMENT

If growth failure is due to a systemic illness, successful treatment of the specific systemic disorder may produce catch-up growth, but severe ill health is more likely to produce permanent stunting. Many relatively 'mild' chronic disorders (e.g. asthma, diabetes) produce delayed puberty (see above) that will eventually show catch-up growth. Improving control in these disorders will often provoke catch-up.

Major systemic disorders that are active in late childhood and early teenage life (e.g. Crohn's disease) reduce the magnitude of the pubertal growth spurt as well as delaying the timing of puberty, and therefore reduce final height. Diseases that affect the skeleton (e.g. rheumatoid arthritis) may produce profound growth failure. Steroid-induced osteoporosis with vertebral fractures, or scoliosis, cause permanent loss of height.

Short stature due to psychosocial deprivation may show impressive catch-up with improved care. Indeed, recovery of height and weight gain (if well documented) while the child is being fostered or is staying in hospital can be used as retrospective evidence in later care proceedings (see Chapter 9).

There is some evidence that a proportion of IUGR children may benefit from a short (2-year) course of GH to induce catch-up growth, although there is currently no licence for this indication in the UK, and further research, especially on longer-term safety, is required before this can be regarded as a routine indication for therapy.

The short and fat child

The main endocrine disorders that cause short stature in children are hypothyroidism, GH deficiency and Cushing's syndrome. Relative obesity is often a feature of all of these conditions. The children may not always appear overweight, but their weight centile is nearer the normal range than their height centile. Skinfold thickness may be increased and derived BMI elevated. There may be a dimpled pattern of centripetal fat distribution (see Figure 4.8).

ACQUIRED HYPOTHYROIDISM

Here there is growth retardation with obesity and usually markedly delayed skeletal maturation and dentition. (Because there is a structural homology between TSH and HCG, prolonged massive elevation of TSH can rarely produce *precocious* puberty in both sexes with lactorrhoea with enlarged testes in the male.)

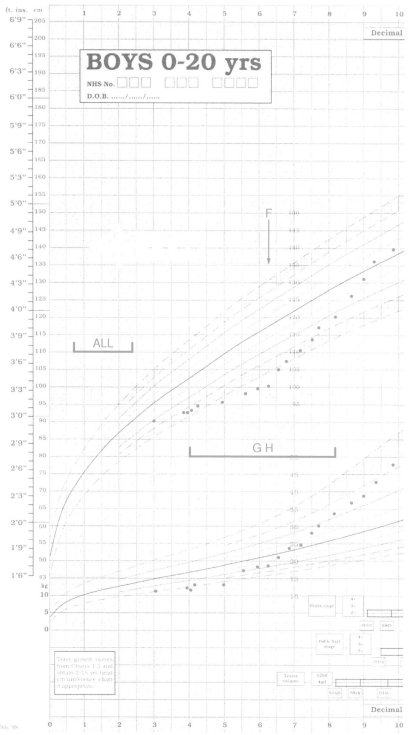

Figure 4.7

Child treated for Acute Lymphoblastic Leukaemia (ALL). Poor growth was noted at follow-up. GH provocation tests showed severe GHD and the child was started on treatment. There was not a good response to GH, possibly due to poor compliance. The child was fostered after their sixth birthday, and this was followed by rapid growth and weight gain. GH status was re-tested at the age of 8 years, with a normal result. GH was then discontinued and good growth was maintained, although excess weight gain required dietary control!

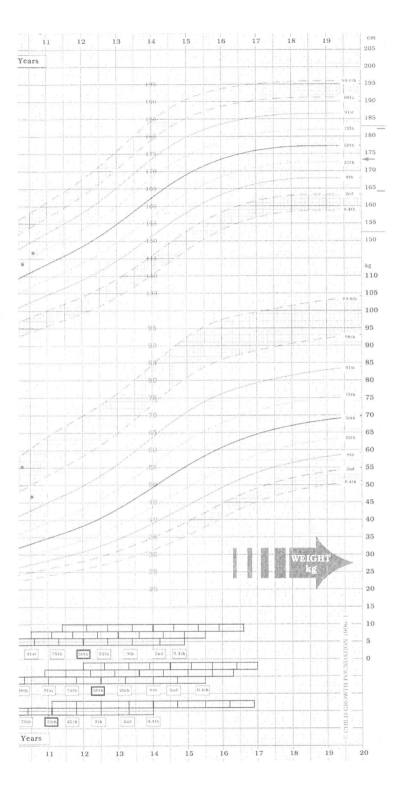

© CHILD GROWTH FOUNDATION 1996/1

Years

cm
205
200
195
190
185
180
175
170
165
160
155
150

kg
110
105
100
95
90
85
80
75
70
65
60
55
50
45
40
35
30
25
20
15
10
5
0

WEIGHT
kg

Years

99.6th
98th
91st
75th
50th
25th
9th
2nd
0.4th

91st 75th 50th 25th 9th 2nd 0.4th

98th 91st 75th 50th 25th 9th 2nd 0.4th

75th 50th 25th 9th 2nd 0.4th

11 12 13 14 15 16 17 18 19 20

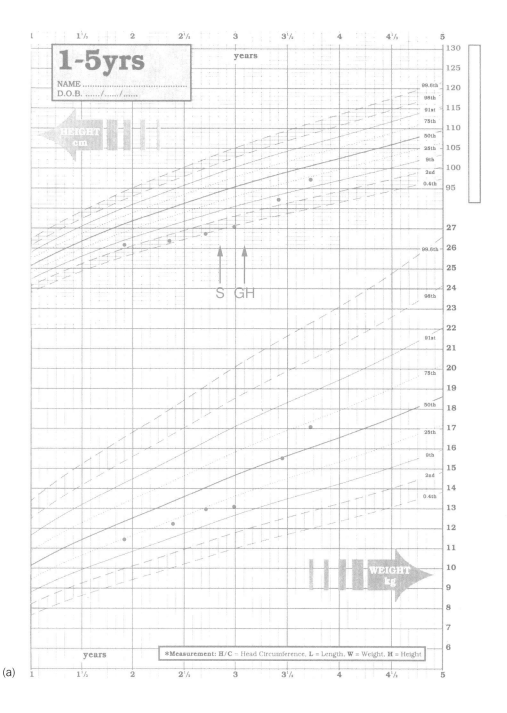

1-5yrs

NAME ....
D.O.B. ..../......./......

years

HEIGHT cm

99.6th
98th
91st
75th
50th
25th
9th
2nd
0.4th

WEIGHT kg

*Measurement: H/C = Head Circumference, L = Length, W = Weight, H = Height

S GH

(a)

Figure 4.8
(a) Evolving craniopharyngioma at presentation and prior to surgery, with subsequent postoperative growth in response to GH and developing obesity secondary to hypothalamic damage. (b) BMI is more than 50% throughout, and skinfolds are also greater than 50%. Contrast with Figure 4.6.

Referral guidelines

Refer a boy whose BMI falls above the 98th centile as obese. Consider referral, as overweight, a boy whose BMI falls above the 91st centile even on the basis of a single measurement. Consider for referral a boy whose BMI falls below the 2nd centile as being significantly underweight even on the basis of a single measurement. During infancy large but transient changes in centile may occur due to the shape of the charts, and these changes are normal. It should be remembered that the earlier the age of the second rise, the greater the risk of future obesity. Remember also that while BMI has a high correlation with relative fatness or leanness it is actually assessing the weight-to-height relationship: **this may give misleading results in boys who are very stocky and muscular who might appear obese on the BMI alone.**

BOYS
BMI CHART
(BIRTH - 20 YEARS)
United Kingdom cross-sectional reference data : 1997/1

Name...

NHS No. ☐☐☐ ☐☐☐ ☐☐☐

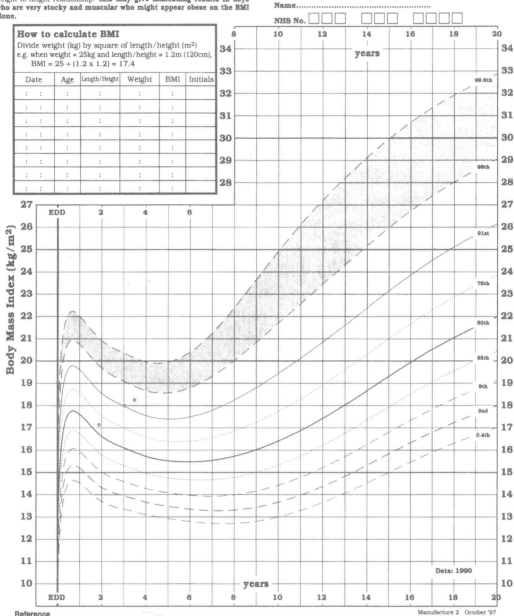

How to calculate BMI
Divide weight (kg) by square of length/height (m²)
e.g. when weight = 25kg and length/height = 1.2m (120cm),
  BMI = 25 ÷ (1.2 x 1.2) = 17.4

Date	Age	Length/Height	Weight	BMI	Initials
: :	:	:	:	:	
: :	:	:	:	:	
: :	:	:	:	:	
: :	:	:	:	:	
: :	:	:	:	:	
: :	:	:	:	:	
: :	:	:	:	:	

(b)

Reference

Body Mass Index reference curves for the UK, 1990 (TJ Cole, JV Freeman, MA Preece) *Arch Dis Child* 1995; **73**: 25-29
Sex differences in weight in infancy (MA Preece, JV Freeman, TJ Cole) *BMJ* 1996; **313**: 1486

Manufacture 2 October '97

Figure 4.8 continued

Most commonly the cause is Hashimoto's disease or autoimmune thyroiditis. It is much commoner in Turner's, Klinefelter's and Down's syndromes, where up to 40% of individuals may be affected. In Down's syndrome there is also an increased incidence of congenital thyroid dysgenesis. Hypothyroidism may also be secondary to rare metabolic disorders such as cystinosis.

As well as a family history of autoimmune disease, there may be a history of tiredness or weakness, constipation, frontotemporal hair loss or dry skin, heat preference and intolerance of cold, deepening of the voice and, in females, menstrual irregularity or long, heavy periods.

On examination there may be goitre, delayed or arrested puberty, myxoedema (rare in childhood), dry skin, vitiligo, hair loss (often in the temporal area), proximal weakness and delayed relaxation of the tendon reflexes (see Figure 4.9).

Congenital hypothyroidism is usually detected by neonatal screening, although in the past when left untreated it was a potent cause of severe short stature.

For the diagnosis of hypothyroidism, serum free T_4 (FT_4) and TSH measurements are most valuable. The combination of a low FT_4 with an elevated TSH concentration is proof of primary hypothyroidism. Antithyroid peroxisomal or microsomal antibodies indicate an autoimmune process in the thyroid, and are usually present in Hashimoto's thyroiditis, as may be antibodies to other glands in the polyendocrinopathy syndromes.

The bone age is often markedly delayed, but catch-up growth may not always occur if the hypothyroid state has been prolonged into the teenage years, as there is often accelerated epiphyseal fusion (see Figure 4.10). After the onset of therapy, weight often decreases markedly.

Figure 4.9
Easy way of demonstrating slowly relaxing reflexes. Ask the child to kneel on a chair and elicit the Achilles tendon reflex. Then observe the time-course of relaxation of the calf muscles. Even in mild hypothyroidism a slow relaxation is obvious.

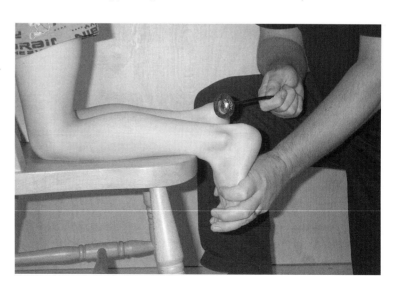

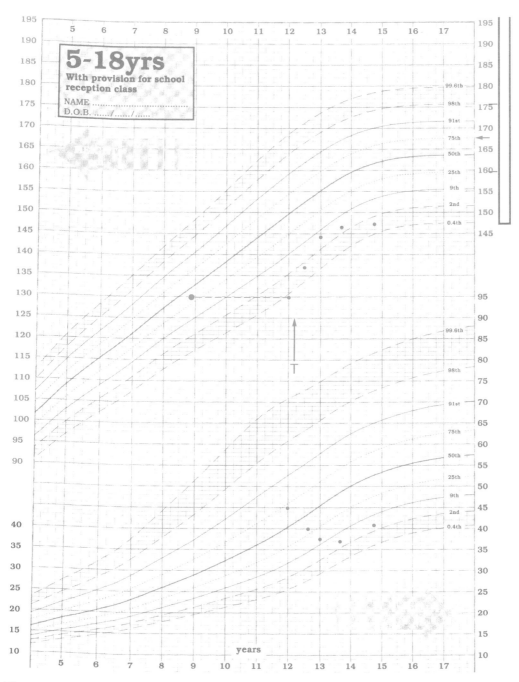

Figure 4.10

Hashimoto's thyroiditis. At presentation this girl was obese with thinning hair, delayed reflexes and a visual field constriction from an enlarged TSH-containing pituitary. Her bone age was delayed by more than 3 years, but on starting treatment she showed a short, sharp growth spurt, menarche at 13¼ years and an eventual reduced final height. She did lose weight and managed to maintain a reasonable BMI at follow-up.

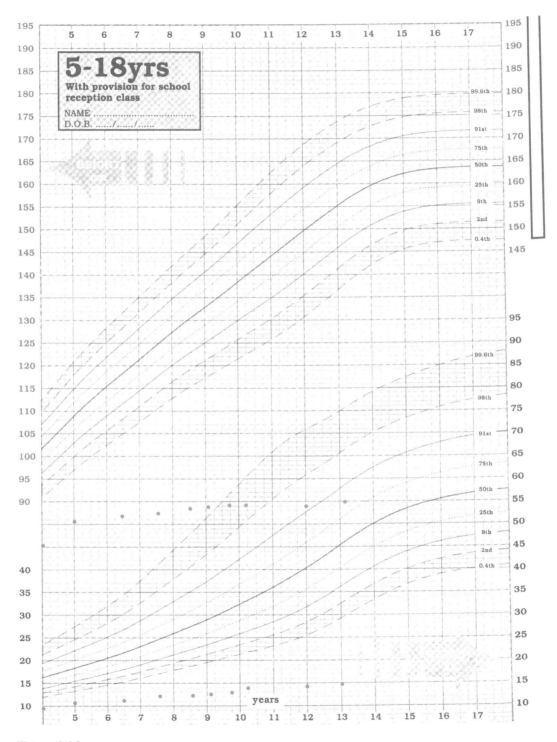

Figure 4.14
Severe syndrome-associated short stature (geleophysic dysplasia). Growth hormone was given between the ages of 6 and 7 years, with no effect.

Some syndromes with chromosomal abnormalities, such as Turner's and Down's syndrome are relatively common (Turner's syndrome has an incidence of 1 in 2500 female births), although of course short stature will not usually be a presenting feature of Down's syndrome. Noonan's syndrome has no known chromosomal basis, and bears a superficial resemblance to Turner's syndrome. It is probably even more common, with some estimates suggesting an incidence as high as 1 in 1000 births.

Turner's syndrome is one of the few syndromic conditions in which the height deficit is potentially remediable. For this reason it will be described in detail and contrasted with Noonan's syndrome.

Most (9 out of 10) Turner's syndrome fetuses do not survive to term, with the majority of losses occurring in the first trimester. The exact chromosomal make-up of the surviving births is very variable, with just over 50% being due to the classical 45XO karyotype and the remainder caused by a variety of mosaics, chromosomal deletions, inversions and rings. Whatever the karyotype, the phenotypic features are similar (including a reduced final height potential), although the likelihood of spontaneous puberty may be greater in the mosaic forms. Rather more XO females will have congenital heart disease. If any Y-chromosome material is present on the karyotype, then gonado-blastoma is a possibility and gonadectomy should be performed.

Nuchal oedema (also present in Down's and other syndromes) may be seen on second-trimester ultrasound scanning and lead to diagnosis on amniocentesis.

Neonatal lymphoedema and the related nail dysplasia may enable an early diagnosis, which should also be suspected in all females with coarctation of the aorta.

The major features of Turner's and Noonan's syndromes are listed in Table 4.5, but it is important to note that up to 40% of girls with Turner's syndrome will show no external features apart from reduced height. *Thus the diagnosis must be suspected in any girl who presents with short stature.*

Final height in Turner's syndrome is reduced by about 18 cm to a mean of around 145–147 cm (depending on the population), but is related to parental height in the same way as in a normal child. There are published centile charts for Turner's and Noonan's syndrome, so a predicted final height may be obtained as described previously (see Figure 4.15).

TREATMENT

GH treatment is licensed for use in Turner's syndrome, and produces an early 'catch-up' phase of growth which may benefit the girl psychologically. The results with regard to final height are less clear-cut, with some studies showing the majority of girls achieving a height within the normal range,

Table 4.5

Differences between Turner's syndrome and Noonan's syndrome

Turner's syndrome	Noonan's syndrome
May have specific learning difficulties; most function well in mainstream education	More likely to have general mild learning difficulty
Left-sided heart defects, coarctation	Right-sided heart abnormalities
99.9% are infertile	Some dominantly inherited, so fertile although boys may have cryptorchidism
45XO or mosaic	Normal chromosomes
Multiple pigmented naevi; conductive hearing loss	Clotting abnormality
All phenotypically female	Male and female

while others are more disappointing, with a mean gain of only 5 cm. These conflicting results may reflect the population in which the Turner's syndrome standards were created, or the population in which the treatment is being administered, as well as differences in ascertainment, timing and dose of adjunctive sex-hormone treatment, or the use of anabolic agents such as oxandrolone. Studies are currently in progress to explore these differences and to try to improve height outcome in all populations.

As well as its licensed indication in Turner's syndrome, the use of GH has also been explored in research trials in Noonan's, Prader–Willi and other syndromes. In these cases the early growth-promoting effects of GH are less pronounced, and final height is not as impressively increased as in GHD, if at all. The potential for side-effects is greater, with some evidence of an increased risk of type 2 diabetes in particular. Treatment outside licence should only be attempted in the context of well-designed clinical studies that are followed through to final height.

The short child with short limbs

There is a spectrum of severity of relatively common short-limbed dwarfing disorders, ranging from the severe, easily recognized achondroplasia to the milder, often undiagnosed hypochondroplasia (see Figures 3.22 and 4.16). The incidence of the severe end of this group of disorders is around 1 in 15 000 live births. Dominant inheritance is the rule, although spontaneous mutations are common. They are caused by a variety of abnormalities of tissue growth factor receptors.

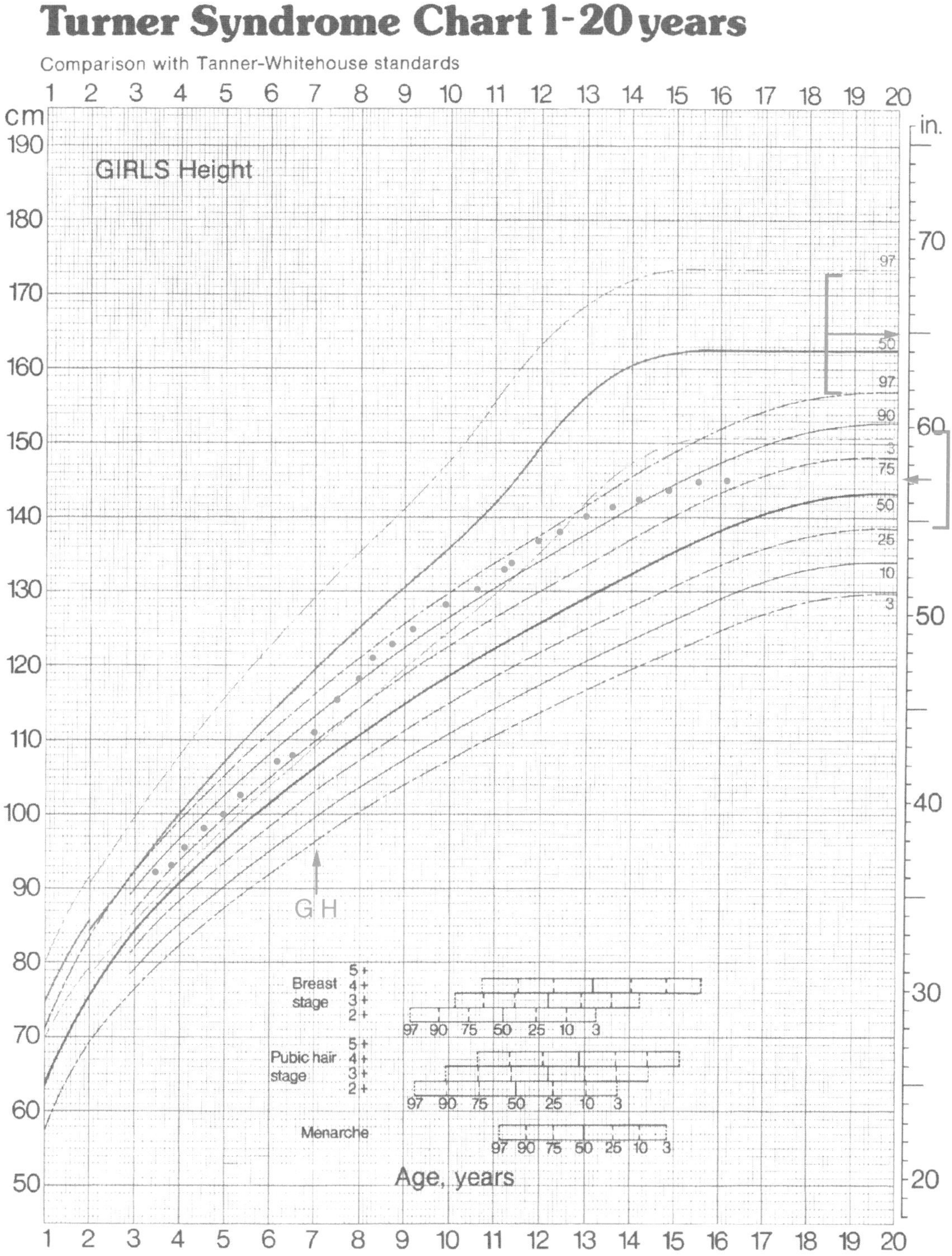

Turner Syndrome Chart 1-20 years

Comparison with Tanner-Whitehouse standards

GIRLS Height

GH

Breast stage 5+ 4+ 3+ 2+
97 90 75 50 25 10 3

Pubic hair stage 5+ 4+ 3+ 2+
97 90 75 50 25 10 3

Menarche
97 90 75 50 25 10 3

Age, years

Figure 4.15

Turner's syndrome and response to GH therapy. The mid-parental height and target centile range are calculated as shown in Figure 3.6. The values are then 'transferred' to the Turner centile range. There is an apparent early response to GH, but little evidence of long-term benefit in this girl who reached spontaneous early puberty at 11¾ years, although oestrogen treatment was eventually required.

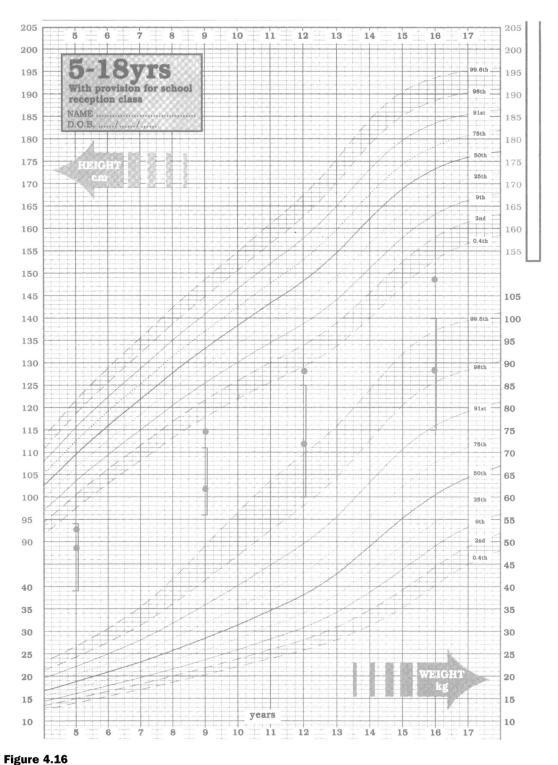

Figure 4.16

Approximate 50th centile ± 2 SD for males with achondroplasia (Horton WA *et al*. (1978) *Journal of Pediatrics* **93**, 435) and the 50th centiles for males with hypochondroplasia (Appan S *et al*. *Acta Paediatrica Scandinavica* **79**, 796).

In the various types of spondyloepiphyseal dysplasia and spondylo-metaphyseal dysplasia (and the combined forms), the spine is affected together with specific areas of the long bones, producing variable shortening of the body segments and spinal deformity. The gait may be abnormal from an early age secondary to coxa vara.

There are also large numbers of specific syndromes with bony dysplasia, some with dysmorphic features which overlap the syndromes mentioned above.

Some metabolic disorders that affect the bone, such as hypo-phosphataemic rickets, may produce limb shortening with bowing of the lower legs.

The diagnosis of these disorders is often difficult, and may require expert radiographic review.

TREATMENT

In the skeletal dysplasias, surgical leg-lengthening techniques in specialist units offer the possibility of height gain of the order of 10–25 cm. (Such techniques have also been used in Turner's syndrome, but with rather less success because of the more common occurrence of contractures. Some cases of idiopathic short stature or late-diagnosed GHD have also been treated in this way.) The technique depends on the creation of an artificial sub-periosteal fracture in the long bones of the leg and upper arm, followed by distraction across the forming callus by external fixation devices that can also correct any angulation that may already exist, or which occurs during the process.

The short-backed child with short stature

This is the rarest group and includes the mucopolysaccharidoses, muco-lipidoses and other storage disorders that may have profound effects on the bony skeleton and other tissues. Many present primarily with neurological signs, although in some disorders, such as Morquio's disease and juvenile Hunter's syndrome, the skeletal features predominate (see Figure 3.22).

Osteogenesis imperfecta and other disorders that affect collagen and fibrin production, such as the Ehlers-Danlos's syndrome, also produce short backs.

Treatment to preserve height is often unsatisfactory. It is highly specialized, and includes bone-marrow transplantation and bisphosphonate therapy.

Investigation of short stature

If the clinical assessment and analysis of the growth curve indicate a pathological growth pattern, further investigations are warranted. In such cases a radiograph of the left hand and wrist for bone age should always be performed (see Chapter 2). Other investigations should be aimed at confirming or ruling out the most likely diagnoses (see Table 4.6).

Table 4.6
Investigation of short stature

Test	Reason
Short and thin	
Full blood count, mean corpuscular volume	Anaemia may be present, especially in inflammatory bowel disease, coeliac disease and renal failure, although it can be present in almost any prolonged illness. Microcytosis is an indication of nutritional deficiency or blood loss, and macrocytosis may indicate malabsorption
Acid–base status, urea and electrolytes, creatinine	Occult renal failure and Bartter's syndrome (hypochloraemic alkalosis). Renal tubular acidosis
Liver function, calcium, phosphate and alkaline phosphatase	Metabolic bone disease and liver disease
Urine analysis (simple biochemistry and microscopy)	Diabetes; renal 'leak'; occult urinary infection
Stool analysis	Giardiasis (produces profound growth retardation and may only be detected if the stool is inspected microscopically for cysts). Fat globules in malabsorption. Reducing substances present in lactose (and rarely other sugar) intolerance. Red blood cells may indicate cow's-milk protein intolerance (CMPI) or coeliac disease and thus the need for a jejunal biopsy
Antigliadin/endomysial antibody screen	Coeliac disease
Chromosome analysis	Turner's syndrome

Short and fat

TSH and FT$_4$	Both are needed – in peripheral hypothyroidism the TSH value will be raised. In hypopituitarism or hypothalamic disease the TSH value may be in the normal range, but inappropriately low for the FT$_4$
IGF-1 and IGFBP-3	May be helpful in confirming diagnosis of GHD (see above). IGF-1 levels are low and GH is normal or high in rare cases of GH insensitivity (e.g. Laron's syndrome)
Lateral skull radiograph	Not a good screening test, but traditionally used to detect enlarged pituitary fossa and/or calcification with craniopharyngioma
Chromosome analysis	Turner's syndrome
GH stimulation test *usually combined with*	GHD
TRH/LHRH tests	For confirmation of hypopituitarism
24-Hour urinary free cortisol (×3)	To exclude Cushing's syndrome

The above may lead on to:

Antithyroid antibodies	Anti-peroxisomal/microsomal antibodies raised in Hashimoto's thyroiditis
MRI	For all cases where GHD (with or without other pituitary hormones) is confirmed
Midnight/9a.m. cortisol	Normal rhythm lost in Cushing's syndrome (midnight level raised). If it is still a possibility, then an overnight dexamethasone suppression test should be considered

Disproportion

Limited skeletal survey (lateral skull, chest, anteroposterior and lateral spine, pelvis and hips, one long bone, bone age)	For specific diagnosis of skeletal dysplasias

Table 4.6 continued

Urine for analysis of mucopolysaccharides, or white-cell enzymes	To exclude mucopolysaccharidoses
Calcium, phosphate and alkaline phosphatase	Metabolic bone diseases (e.g. hypophosphataemic rickets)
White-cell enzyme levels	For other storage disorders (especially if full blood count shows vacuolated lymphocytes)

Psychological problems related to short stature

For some patients, even relatively modest short stature is an overwhelming perceived cause for concern in their life. I have received letters from male adults of moderate normal height (e.g. 172 cm) telling of their distress, to the extent of attempted suicide, about being 'too short'. Other individuals who are well below 4 SD from the mean have no concerns at all, other than those related to accompanying pathology, infertility, etc.

The extremely short individual may have physical difficulties in finding comfortable seating, reaching light switches, etc., and those with short-limbed dysplasias experience additional problems with tampon insertion, bottom-wiping, etc. For these reasons, late leg/arm lengthening may be considered in some cases.

Children with secondary short stature may obviously have problems that are directly related not to their size, but to their other pathology.

Patients who have been referred because of idiopathic short stature represent a selected group, and there is some evidence of under-achievement at school, socially and professionally. Conversely, there is ample evidence that society favours tallness (e.g. US bishops are taller than curates, the taller presidential candidate more often wins the election than might be expected by chance, in mock job interviews there is evidence of prejudice towards the taller candidates, etc.). However, the problems related to short stature in an unselected population of short individuals are less easy to document. There is no good evidence of extra bullying or under-performance either in child-hood or in later life.

There are several excellent support groups for short people (see Appendix), which provide information, peer support and professional training.

- other rarer syndromes;
- genetic disorders of enzyme production that cause sex steroid deficiency;
- pure gonadal dysgenesis (defective germ cell migration);
- complete androgen insensitivity.

Acquired primary gonadal failure may be seen in the following:

- autoimmune disorders;
- galactosaemia;
- post-infections (e.g. mumps);
- damage from irradiation to the gonad and some chemotherapy regimes;
- trauma, either *in utero* or later torsion.

Hypogonadotropic hypogonadism

This is associated with the following:

- temporary deficiency, associated with delayed maturation, chronic illnesses and systemic diseases, stress, anorexia, over-training and malnutrition;
- hypothyroidism;
- isolated (with anosmia = Kallmann's syndrome; other rarer syndromes);
- hypopituitarism.

Thereafter, tests will depend on whether one is dealing with hyper- or hypogonadotropism.

Tests indicated in hypergonadotropic hypogonadism

These are as follows:

- karyotype (it may sometimes be necessary to take both blood and fibroblast specimens to exclude tissue mosaicism);
- urinary adrenal steroid profile to exclude disorders of testosterone synthesis;
- pelvic ultrasonography for ovarian or uterine morphology, or to locate impalpable testes. Laparoscopy may then be needed to assess the possibility of orchidopexy or the need for gonadectomy to prevent undetected malignant change of the testes;

- if the LH/FSH levels are borderline, or in prepubertal individuals in whom damage is a possibility, then a human chorionic gonadotropin (HCG) test can be performed. This stimulates production of oestrogen or testosterone that can be measured as a rise from the basal values, which provides information about possible gonadal function in cases where there is mild, compensated hypogonadism;
- autoantibodies to the thyroid, adrenal and ovary can be estimated in the presence of a family history or suggestive physical signs.

Tests indicated in hypogonadotropic hypogonadism

These are as follows:

- LHRH test to check presence of gonadotropins – an FSH rise to > 2.6 is said to exclude hypogonadotropism;
- thyroid function;
- other pituitary hormones, especially prolactin;
- MRI scan to image the pituitary and hypothalamus if there is anything other than simple delay.

Therapy for delayed puberty

Simple delay in males is treated with testosterone. This may either be given in a depot dosage of 50 or 100 mg of testosterone esters (Sustanon) every 3–4 weeks intramuscularly, or as oral testosterone undecanoate, 20–40 mg per day. An alternative approach, especially in younger patients, is to use the anabolic steroid oxandrolone at a dose of 1.25–2.5 mg per day orally. Usually these treatments are discontinued after 3 or 4 months, and the development of testicular size after cessation of treatment (which will suppress testicular growth) is checked together with serum testosterone measurements. If puberty starts (testicular volume > 4 mL), no more treatment is required and natural puberty should progress (see Figure 4.4).

If there is failure of subsequent development, a further 3-month course and re-evaluation of the possibility of permanent central hypogonadism may be necessary. Permanent lifelong treatment to protect the cardiovascular system and preserve bone mineral density may be required. If there is testicular damage then infertility is likely and testicular prostheses can be inserted for cosmetic reasons. However, modern IVF techniques may allow fertility from even a few aspirated sperm, so it is worth attempting to preserve externally palpable testicular remnants.

In females, pubertal delay requiring treatment is less common but may be treated with low doses of oestradiol (in ng/kg doses) by patch or orally, usually for 3–4 months as in the male, after which spontaneous puberty continues. The dose is gradually increased over 2–3 years to an adult HRT dose if there is permanent deficiency, in order to induce breast development, prevent osteoporosis and ensure normal psychosocial development. Counselling about infertility and the possible need for IVF may be required.

Further reading

Brook CGD (ed.) (2001) *Clinical paediatric endocrinology*, 4th edn. Blackwell Science, Oxford.

Buckler JMH (1987) *The adolescent years*. Castlemead Publications, Ware.

Buckler JMH (1994) *Growth disorders in children*. BMJ Publishing, London.

Wales JKH, Wit JM and Rogol AD (1996) *A color atlas of pediatric endocrinology and growth*. Mosby-Wolfe, London.

Tall stature

History

As with cases of short stature, determine what it is that is concerning the parents – and the patient if he or she is old enough – as well as the referring health professional. Many parents have concerns about their normal, genetically tall child based on their own social experiences of being tall. The emphasis of the history is often quite different to that used to assess short stature.

Note: in the following, items marked* are found in several dysmorphic syndromes associated with short stature.

The history should cover the following:

- birth size – weight, length and occipitofrontal circumference if recorded (birth weight has only a poor predictive value for subsequent height, but in some rare causes of later tallness, birth size is substantially increased over that which might be expected genetically);
- mode of delivery – large babies born to small mothers are at risk of shoulder dystocia;
- growth rate in height – as recorded in past medical records or by the parents ('Are they shooting up much faster than their friends?');
- weight changes – sudden weight gain or loss;
- family heights – (preferably measured directly; see Chapter 2). Do any parents, siblings or more distant relatives have noticeably tall stature?
- parental build – thin or heavy;
- age of menarche in mother;
- post-menarchal patient – irregular, light or heavy periods;
- sexual maturation of father – in relation to his peers (voice breaking or shaving);
- parental consanguinity – increased risk of autosomal recessive disorders;

- family ill health – autoimmune problems, 'gland disorders', early heart disease or eye operations (Marfan's syndrome);
- development – school problems (various syndromes*), including anxiety/ fidgeting/odd behaviour (thyrotoxicosis);
- loose stools, palpitations, diplopia, heat intolerance – thyrotoxicosis;
- secondary sex characteristics – body odour, greasy hair, acne, moodiness, vaginal discharge, hairiness, breast development;
- sense of smell – anosmia in hypogonadotropic hypogonadism;
- drugs – anabolic agents, the 'pill';
- diet – obesity;
- oestrogenic compounds – phyto-oestrogens (e.g. soya/cannabis, and used in some foods as fattening agents in meat industry).

Examination

The examination should include the following:

- weight in relation to height:
  thin – Marfan's syndrome, thyrotoxicosis;
  fat – obesity;
- disproportion (long legs) – Marfan's syndrome, hypogonadism;
- raised occipitofrontal circumference – Sotos' syndrome;
- dysmorphic features – various syndromes*;
- hand:
  deep-set nails – Sotos' syndrome;
  sweaty plus tremor – thyrotoxicosis;
  hyper-mobility of the fingers/wrist *plus*
      long, thin fingers (arachnodactyly) *plus*
      long span – Marfan's syndrome;
- eyes:
  exophthalmos/chemosis – thyrotoxicosis;
  visual field defects – pituitary adenomas;
  lens dislocation (up) – Marfan's syndrome;
  lens dislocation (down) – homocystinuria;
  high arched palate – Marfan's syndrome;
- thyroid (goitre):
  palpation from behind the patient to measure size and shape of the gland, which should move upwards on swallowing;
  irregularity and lymph nodes – adenomas and carcinoma, as in MEN 2b (multiple endocrine neoplasia type 2b with Marfanoid habitus and medullary carcinoma);
  bruit – thyrotoxicosis;

- blood pressure elevated – 11β-hydroxylase form of congenital adrenal hyperplasia;
- heart murmur (aortic/mitral incompetence) – Marfan's syndrome;
- tachycardia, wide pulse pressure – thyrotoxicosis;
- pectus excavatum or pectus carinatum – Marfan's syndrome;
- back:
  horizontal striae – rapid growth from any cause;
  scoliosis – Marfan's syndrome;
- abdominal organomegaly – neonate with Beckwith–Wiedemann's syndrome (where an umbilical hernia or omphalocoele can also be seen);
- abdominal/pelvic mass – tumours with sex-hormone production;
- gynaecomastia:
  true – Klinefelter's syndrome, hypogonadism;
  mimicked – obesity;
- muscularity increased – non-salt-losing males with congenital adrenal hyperplasia; anabolic steroid abuse;
- hemihypertrophy/overgrowth – Beckwith–Wiedemann's syndrome;
- skin:
  lacy-edged *café-au-lait* spot – McCune–Albright's syndrome (with sexual precocity and bone lesions);
- striae (breast/abdomen) – obesity;
- hair loss – thyrotoxicosis;
- pubertal staging (see Chapter 4):
  looking for precocity – in particular look for concordance or discordance of features (see Chapter 7);
  small hard testes – Klinefelter's syndrome;
  small soft testes – congenital adrenal hyperplasia, anabolic steroids;
- CNS:
  anxiety/psychosis – thyrotoxicosis;
  brisk reflexes – thyrotoxicosis.

An algorithm can be used to aid diagnosis in tall stature (see Figure 6.1).

Idiopathic or genetic tall stature is by far the commonest cause of concern about excess height.

There are a relatively small number of primary syndromes of large size with or without learning difficulties.

Secondary causes of increased final height are rare, although some secondary conditions produce largeness only for a period of the child's growth span, and then a normal or even reduced final height if early bony fusion occurs.

There are some very rare primary disorders of blood supply or pathology intrinsic to the growth plate that can produce localized overgrowth, but which are not associated with overall tall stature.

Figure 6.1
Diagnostic algorithm for tall
stature.

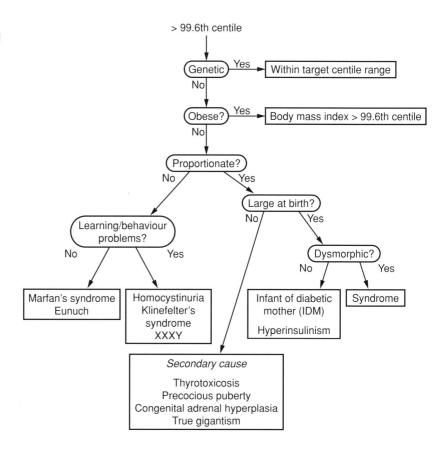

Idiopathic tall stature

This is defined by the absence of abnormalities in the history and physical examination, except for commonly horizontal striae on the back after a period of rapid growth. It is usually familial, with tall stature throughout childhood and an increased final height. The height velocity varies around the 75th centile (see Chapter 3). The final height is within the range defined by parental size (see Chapter 3). The bone age approximates to chronological age, and there is a normal age of onset of puberty. In constitutional early puberty there will be a moderately advanced bone age (not more than +2 SD above chronological age) with an increased height velocity (>75%) in the later childhood years and early onset and cessation of puberty, often following the same pattern as one or both of the parents. A combination of the two patterns is not uncommon (see Figure 6.2).

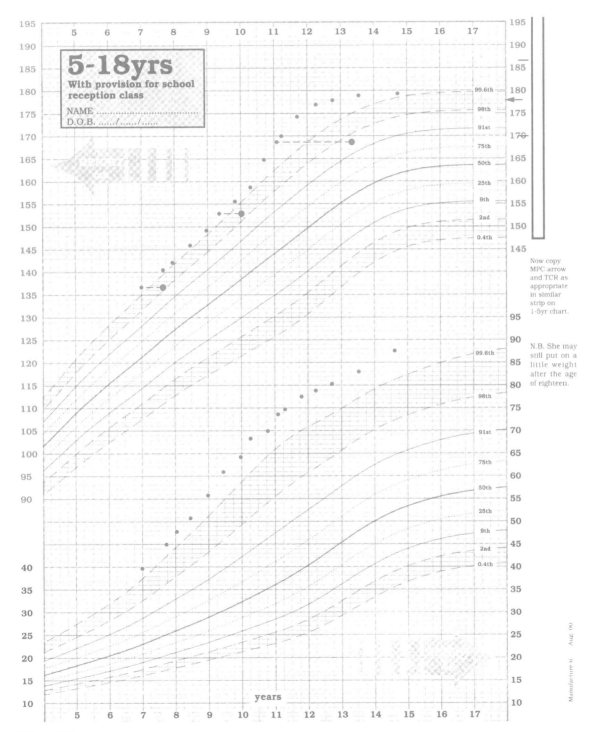

Figure 6.2
Constitutional tall stature with slightly early puberty, probably enhanced by being moderately overweight.

Other primary causes of tall stature

These may be subdivided as follows.

PROPORTIONATE LARGE SIZE WITH INTELLECTUAL DEFICIT

There are a few rare syndromes associated with tall stature and mental retardation, such as Sotos', Weaver's and Marshall–Smith's syndromes. In Sotos' syndrome the head is disproportionately large, the child is clumsy, with variable learning difficulty, and the fingernails are deep-set.

Beckwith–Wiedemann's syndrome with neonatal macrosomia and hypoglycaemia with organomegaly, macroglossia and umbilical hernia/omphalocoele is caused by a relative excess of insulin-like growth factor 2 (IGF-2) *in utero* due to an imprinting defect. Intellectual deficit may occur as a result of the hypoglycaemia, but if this is avoided intellectual development is usually normal.

DISPROPORTIONATE TALL STATURE WITH NORMAL INTELLECT

Marfan's syndrome is a relatively common dominantly inherited disorder characterized by disproportionate tall stature (see Figure 3.22). There are many children with some of the features of the condition, but because of the important genetic and cardiac implications it should only be diagnosed if the following criteria are met (see Box 6.1).

Box 6.1   Features of Marfan's syndrome (major features are indicated by bold typeface)

Skeletal	**Long span. Long legs compared to the back, arachnodactyly, joint laxity, scoliosis and chest deformities. High arched palate.** Flat feet
Eyes	Myopia, **lens dislocation** or poor fixation of the lens, flat cornea and hypoplastic iris
CVS	Mitral and aortic valve incompetence, **aortic dilatation and dissection**
Chest	Spontaneous pneumothorax
Skin	Herniae, striae
MRI spine	**Lumbosacral dural ectasia**

If there is no family history there should be at least two major features in two systems, with involvement in one other system. If the family history is positive (with or without proven abnormality of the fibrillin gene), then one major feature plus involvement in one other system allows the diagnosis.

Hypogonadism can cause a modestly increased final height with long legs (the so-called 'eunuchoid body habitus'). This is due to late closure of the epiphyses and prolonged childhood growth of the legs, coupled with failure of the sex-hormone-mediated growth of the spine (see Chapter 1 and Figure 3.22). The X-linked Kallmann's syndrome of hypogonadotropic hypogonadism is associated with moderately tall stature and anosmia.

DISPROPORTIONATE TALL STATURE PLUS INTELLECTUAL DEFICIT

Sex chromosome abnormalities

Klinefelter's syndrome (XXY, XXYY, XXXY and mosaic forms) and the XYY syndromes produce tallness, and both the legs are relatively long compared to the back. (Other abnormalities involving duplication of the X- or Y-chromosomes may occur, but are associated with normal or short stature.)

Klinefelter's syndrome is most commonly associated with the XXY karyotype, but variants with XXYY and mosaic forms can occur. There tend to be behavioural and learning problems of varying degree. There will be small, firm testes which may be mal-descended, and hypergonadotrophic hypogonadism. The infertility can sometimes be treated with advanced IVF techniques such as intra-cytoplasmic sperm injection (ICSI). There is often gynaecomastia, and there is an increased risk of diabetes mellitus in later life.

XYY males have a mild intellectual deficit and specific motor co-ordination problems, but normal behaviour. This syndrome is no longer thought to be associated with psychopathic tendencies. Cryptorchidism occurs, but not as commonly as in Klinefelter's syndrome.

Homocystinuria

This is an aminoaciduria that is associated with marfanoid tall stature, but will much more frequently present because of the associated learning difficulties and eye problems (ectopia lentis and severe myopia), rather than because of tall stature *per se*. Late thromboembolic and cardiovascular problems occur. Diagnosis can be confirmed by measuring plasma homocystine levels.

Secondary causes of tall stature

EARLY ONSET

Intrauterine hyperinsulinaemia, either due to primary inherited disorders of pancreatic beta-cell function, or secondary to second/third trimester hyperglycaemia due to maternal diabetes, causes early macrosomia as insulin is a potent fetal growth factor. Once the abnormal insulin-secreting environment is removed after birth there is 'catch-down' growth to normal genetic centiles by 2 years of age (see Figure 6.3). Infants of diabetic mothers have a characteristic phenotype and also an increased incidence of congenital malformations whose risk is related to periconceptional control and HbA_{1c} levels.

LATE ONSET

The commonest cause by far is tall stature due to nutritional obesity (see Chapter 7). In childhood, excess calorie intake is made available for growth, and raises IGF-1 levels thus producing relatively tall stature characterized by a height at the upper end of the predicted target range. Puberty often occurs relatively early, and final height is therefore only modestly increased. There is often a similar history and body shape in one or both parents and in the siblings. Hypothalamic brain tumours may very rarely produce pathological overeating and secondary tall stature, but in such cases there are usually obvious CNS symptoms and signs.

Other causes of large size are rare. They include pituitary gigantism and thyrotoxicosis (sexual precocity is dealt with separately in Chapter 7).

Pituitary gigantism is *extremely* rare. Growth hormone excess is usually secondary to a GH-producing adenoma in the pituitary, either *de novo* or secondary to McCune–Albright syndrome, and is equivalent to acromegaly, but occurring before epiphyseal fusion. As in acromegaly there may be prognathism and signs of optic chiasm compression. The tall stature is proportionate with an elevated height velocity (see Figure 6.4).

Thyrotoxicosis, if relatively mild (and hence unrecognized and untreated), produces an acceleration of growth rate and relative tall stature in mid-childhood, although there is an advanced bone age and the eventual height is only mildly elevated (see Figure 6.5). It is almost always caused by Graves' disease and the presence of thyroid-stimulating antibodies, as in the adult population. Eye disease is usually less pronounced in children than in adults. It is very much more common in females and like other autoimmune diseases, is strongly familial.

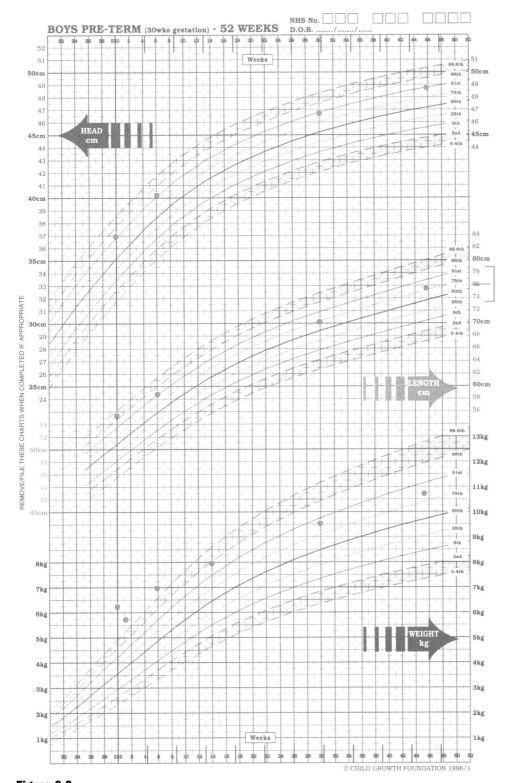

Figure 6.3
'Catch-down' growth of infant of diabetic mother. There was shoulder dystocia causing a severe Erb's palsy.

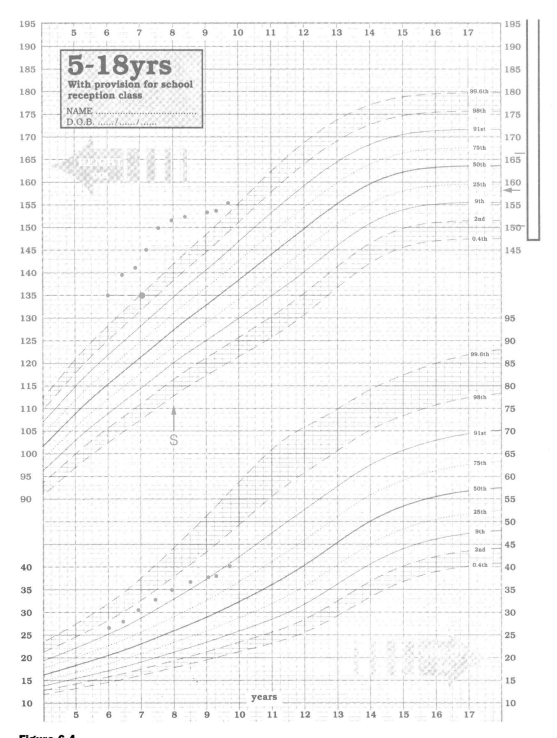

Figure 6.4
True gigantism before and after pituitary surgery. If left untreated, heights in excess of 240 cm have been recorded.

Investigation of tall stature

A hand and wrist radiograph for bone age will serve the dual purpose of providing an estimation of physiological maturity and allowing quantification of arachnodactyly by estimation of the metacarpal index (see Figure 6.6), as well as showing certain semi-specific abnormalities in some of the rare overgrowth syndromes.

A metacarpal index compares the average length to width ratios of the metacarpal bones in an attempt to define arachnodactyly as a value of > 8.5.

If Marfan's syndrome is suspected, then a cardiac ultrasound examination should be performed. If the patient does not have enough 'points' on the Marfan scoring system (see above) for the condition, and a normal ultrasound, then they may be reassured that they do not have the full condition.

If there are any genital abnormalities or behavioural or learning difficulties, the karyotype should be checked. In boys with Klinefelter's syndrome, the primary testicular damage will produce menopausal LH levels.

Hypothalamic or pituitary hypogonadism will produce hypogonadotropism, and the LH and FSH levels will also be suppressed by peripheral testosterone production or anabolic steroid administration.

The diagnosis of thyrotoxicosis is confirmed by high (F)T_4 levels in the presence of suppressed TSH levels. Hypothyroidism is a rare cause of sexual precocity, and the TSH level will be grossly elevated.

If pituitary gigantism is a possibility, then an elevated IGF-1 level may be a useful screening test, followed by a GH suppression test (in response to an oral glucose tolerance test the GH level should become undetectable), and pituitary MRI imaging performed in a specialized unit.

Therapy for tall stature

Very few children require treatment for tall stature. None of the therapies is without risk, and their use always should be confined to experienced centres.

Arbitrary definitions of 'excessive' final height can be made (i.e. more than 185 cm in a girl or 200 cm in a boy), although much depends on the population mean height, the psychological adjustment of the child, and support from the child's parents and peers. The child him- or herself (not just the parents – one of whom may have had bad experiences related to tall stature in their youth) should request treatment and understand the potential risks involved.

Induction of accelerated puberty by administering high daily doses of oral ethinyloestradiol (100–200 µg) to girls or depot injections of testosterone

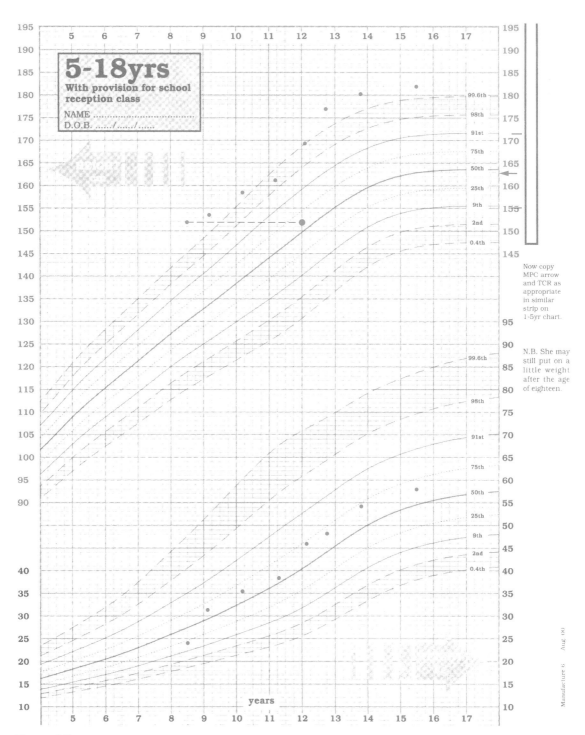

Figure 6.5
Height in thyrotoxicosis: tall and thin at presentation, but with a final height above the top end of the TCR.

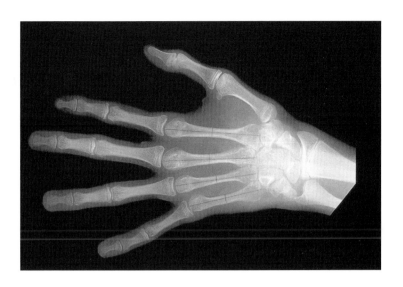

Figure 6.6
Hand and wrist X-ray for bone age and metacarpal index.

(up to 500 mg every 2 weeks) to boys will limit final height *if started early in puberty.* The sudden onset of sexual maturity may produce behavioural problems. Girls may develop tender breasts with striae, and boys may develop priapism. Both may develop acne. Serious short-term risks have been described, especially thromboembolism, with high-dose oestrogen treatment, and the unquantifiable risks of long-term side-effects are a cause for concern. It would probably be unwise to treat girls in families with a strong history of thromboembolism or breast cancer.

Surgical drilling of the epiphyses of the femur and tibia can produce arrest of leg growth (and minimal scarring) in the hands of an experienced paediatric orthopaedic surgeon.

Associated treatments

Boys with Klinefelter's syndrome and other hypogonadal males need testosterone replacement therapy in order to undergo sexual development as well as bony fusion to limit height and minimize body disproportion. Depot testosterone (50–100–250 mg injections), slowly increased from a time compatible with the development of the child's peers, is commonly used. Patch therapy may become more acceptable in the near future. Long-term oral treatment is not usually recommended because of the potential for hepatic side-effects. Exogenous testosterone may worsen pre-existing behavioural problems.

Hypogonadal girls can be treated with oestrogen orally or by patch.

THYROTOXICOSIS

For individuals with thyrotoxicosis there are three therapies that can be used sequentially or individually, although all of them should be confined to specialist centres. In some cases, as well as stimulating antibodies there are also antithyroid antibodies, in which case spontaneous hypothyroidism may ensue after initial toxicosis – so-called 'Hashitoxicosis'. It is therefore often worth undertaking a trial of drug therapy before starting 'definitive' treatment in the hope of remission, especially if antithyroid antibodies are present in high titre.

Antithyroid drugs

Propylthiouracil (PTU), methimazole and carbimazole can be given at a dose sufficient to suppress thyroid function, with or without added thyroxine to maintain euthyroidism. The duration of treatment is 6 months to 2 years, and remission is achieved in about 50% of cases.

The disadvantages of this form of therapy are the long duration of treatment, problems with compliance, and the risk of toxic side-effects (agranulocytosis in particular).

For initial symptomatic relief, in addition to antithyroid therapies for the first 4–6 weeks, beta-blockers (usually propranolol) can be used. These provide rapid symptomatic relief, but cannot be used if there is a history of asthma.

If relapse occurs, antithyroid therapy may be resumed or the patient may be offered the choice of surgical or radio-iodine therapy.

(Sub)-total thyroidectomy

Occasionally this may be used as a first-line therapy. It is more commonly used in cases of relapse. The advantages of this form of therapy are that it is usually a 'one-off' treatment. The disadvantages are as follows:

- it requires a surgeon experienced in childhood operation;
- permanent hypothyroidism (majority of cases);
- permanent hypoparathyroidism (rare);
- damage to the recurrent laryngeal nerve.

Iodine[131] treatment

This may occasionally be used as a first-line therapy. However, it is more commonly used in cases of relapse. Although it is effective in the majority of cases, the disadvantages include later hypothyroidism (20% < 1 year; 60% < 10 years) and the possible risk of later malignant change (probably very small or zero).

Psychosocial aspects of tall stature

Pathological causes of tall stature are relatively common. For instance, Klinefelter's syndrome occurs more than twice as frequently as Turner's syndrome in birth karyotype surveys. However, the social acceptability of tall stature means that far fewer cases are referred for assessment.

Some individuals are extremely concerned about 'standing out from a crowd' and are worried about finding a partner. Late limb reduction surgery may sometimes be offered but is rarely successful. A tall parent may have (often unfounded) concerns about the ability of their children to accept their tallness. The support groups for tall people (see Appendix) provide help and advice, including practical matters such as how to find large clothes and shoes.

Further reading

Brook CGD (ed.) (2001) *Clinical paediatric endocrinology*, 4th edn. Blackwell Science, Oxford.

Hochberg Z (1999) *Practical algorithms in paediatric endocrinology*. Karger, Basel.

Kelnar CJH, Savage MO, Stirling HF and Saegner P (eds) (1998) *Growth disorders – pathophysiology and treatment*. Chapman and Hall, London.

Wales JKH, Wit JM and Rogol AD (1996) *A color atlas of pediatric endocrinology and growth*. Mosby-Wolfe, London.

Early sexual development

Introduction

Early or precocious puberty (PP) is defined as the onset of puberty before 8 years (in girls) or 9 years (in boys). It can be subdivided into 'true' (or 'central') precocious puberty and 'pseudo' sexual precocity.

In central precocious puberty all of the events of normal puberty occur early, but with their normal temporal relationship.

In pseudoprecocious puberty only some aspects of sexual development occur, secondary to androgen or oestrogen production in the periphery. It can be sub-classified into isosexual precocity (i.e. oestrogen in the female, testosterone in the male) or heterosexual precocity (i.e. oestrogen production in the male or testosterone production in the female).

Finally, there are two forms of partial development, which may be regarded as variations of normality, namely premature adrenarche and premature thelarche.

Note: as the first sign of true precocious puberty in a girl is breast development, the differentiation between early puberty and premature thelarche cannot be made only on the basis of a single physical examination. One must consider both growth pattern and bone age – which are normal in premature thelarche and accelerated in precocious puberty.

Causes of true sexual precocity

These include the following:

● idiopathic causes – by far the most frequent form, most common in girls;
● CNS abnormalities – most common in boys (congenital anomalies, hypothalamic hamartomas, elevated intracranial pressure, or tumours);
● cranial irradiation – especially low doses (1800 cGy) in girls;
● hypothyroidism – longstanding, untreated (caused by a cross-reaction of TSH with the gonadotropin receptor).

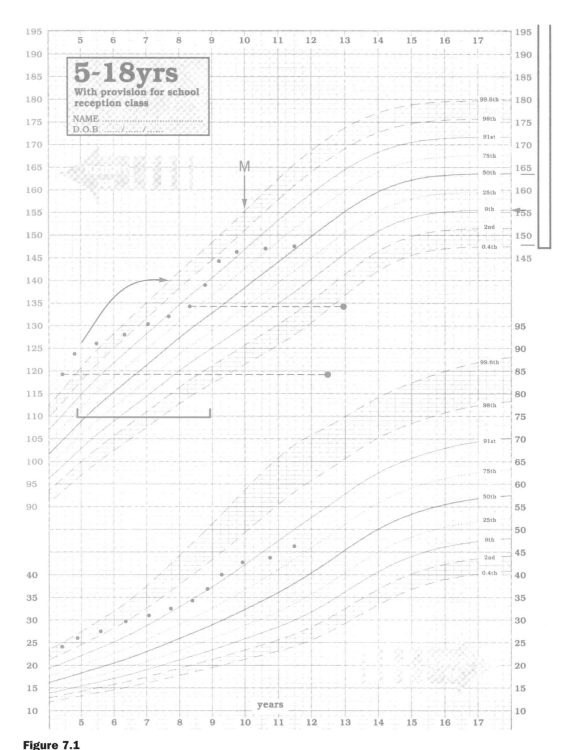

Figure 7.1
Precocious puberty due to hamartoma of the base of the brain (tuber cinereum). Tall with bone age advanced by 7.5 years at presentation. Arrow shows the likely untreated course and final height of 140 cm. Treatment with a gonadotropin-releasing hormone analogue was continued for 4 years, during which time bone age only advanced by 0.5 years. After discussion, treatment was discontinued at the age of 9 years, with menarche at 10 years and a final height of 148 cm (bottom end of genetic range).

> **Box 7.1** True sexual precocity (or central precocious puberty)
>
> Concordant pubertal development (i.e. stage 3 breasts and pubic hair + uterine and ovarian maturation, or testes 12 mL + stage 3 penis and pubic hair)
>
> *plus* secondary mood swings, acne, body odour, vaginal discharge, etc.
>
> *plus* height spurt with advanced bone age leading to premature epiphyseal closure and reduced final height (see Figure 5.6)

Causes of pseudosexual precocity

These include the following:

- adrenal tumours – testosterone or oestrogen;
- non-salt-losing congenital adrenal hyperplasia – testosterone;
- exogenous sex steroid administration – contraceptive pill, anabolic steroids;
- gonadal tumours – oestrogen or testosterone;
- gonadotropin or human chorionic gonadotropin-producing tumours – liver, testis;
- ovarian cysts – oestrogen-secreting;
- McCune–Albright syndrome (an activating mutation of an ubiquitous endocrine receptor) – lacy-edged *café-au-lait* patches with or without bony dysplasia, often discordant pubertal changes;
- testotoxicosis – familial, male pseudoprecocious puberty; testes are often relatively small.

> **Box 7.2** Pseudosexual precocity
>
> | Feature | Comments |
> |---|---|
> | Target tissue + + | (Breast hypertrophy in oestrogen excess; cliteromegaly + pubic hair in heterosexual and penis + pubic hair in isosexual androgen excess) |
> | Testes/ovary suppressed | Small soft testes; ovaries non-follicular and low volume on ultrasound scan |
> | Advanced bone age Accelerated growth rate (see Figure 4.3) | |

Variations of normality

Box 7.3   Premature adrenarche

Pubic and axillary hair, acne, body odour, mildly advanced bone age, and no or only mild acceleration of height velocity.

Adrenarche is a normal age-related maturation of the adrenal cortex with increased secretion of androgenic precursors of testosterone, namely androstenedione and particularly dehydroepiandrosterone sulphate (DHEAS). It usually merges into normal puberty, but if markedly early maturation occurs, then the mild androgenic effects are noticeable, particularly in females. It may occasionally be familial or secondary to intracranial pathology. There is some evidence that an inherited adrenal enzyme over-activity causes the condition in some cases. It has a tendency to 'evolve' in teenage life into a polycystic ovarian (PCO) phenotype with dys-menorrhoea, hirsutism, insulin resistance and obesity.

Box 7.4   Premature thelarche

Early breast enlargement, usually in infancy, and often cyclical with no other pubertal changes, and normal or only mildly advanced growth and skeletal maturation (see Figure 7.2).

Thelarche is common and usually presents as isolated bi- or uni-lateral breast enlargement in infancy. The breasts may vary in size but do not progressively enlarge and there are no other signs of puberty.

Investigation of early sexual development

Previous records of height allow estimation of accelerated growth rate. A bone age will give information about the progress towards epiphyseal fusion.

Together with accurate documentation of all signs of puberty, in girls pelvic and abdominal ultrasound examination for ovary and uterine size (and in both sexes to exclude sex-hormone-producing tumours and to estimate adrenal size) allows assessment of the likely cause and the extent to which any changes have progressed.

Measurement of testosterone and/or oestradiol (E_2), coupled with measurement of the gonadotropins LH and FSH (either basal or in response to gonadotropin-releasing-hormone stimulation), differentiates between true

Treatment

For true precocious puberty, because of the likely reduced final height and psychological problems, treatment is usually offered in specialist units. Treatment in girls over 7 years of age is neither effective nor usually warranted. Depot slow-release luteinizing-hormone-releasing hormone (LHRH) analogues administered intramuscularly or subcutaneously every 4–12 weeks through local anaesthetic are commonly used. These abolish cyclical gonadotropin production by the pituitary and hence suppression of sexual development. Initially this is combined with the oral sex-steroid synthesis blocker, cyproterone acetate, to prevent the early hyperstimulation by the agonist. Treatment is continued until the final height prediction has become acceptable and the child's peer group is showing pubertal changes. There are no long-term recognized side-effects, and the suppression is reversible on stopping treatment.

Gonadotropin-independent precocity will not, by definition, respond to LHRH analogue treatment, and therefore steroid synthesis blockers may be used, although there may be side-effects and treatment is often not as effective unless it is amenable to surgical intervention. Non-salt-losing congenital adrenal hyperplasia is treated with steroid replacement. Adrenarche is benign (although later polycystic ovarian syndrome (PCO) may supervene; see above), and thelarche requires no intervention.

Further reading

Brook CGD (ed.) (2001) *Clinical paediatric endocrinology*, 4th edn. Blackwell Science, Oxford.

Kelnar CJH, Savage MO, Stirling HF and Saegner P (eds) (1998) *Growth disorders – pathophysiology and treatment*. Chapman and Hall, London.

Wales JKH, Wit JM and Rogol AD (1996) *A color atlas of pediatric endocrinology and growth*. Mosby-Wolfe, London.

Obesity

For the first time in the history of the world, the number of people affected by diseases of affluence now outstrips the number affected by starvation. In the UK, as in most of the developed world, there is a steady increase in the weight for age of the childhood population, and in the number of children referred for their obesity. There are also increasing numbers of children presenting with what are classically regarded as 'adult' diseases, such as type 2 diabetes, as a consequence of their obesity. In addition, there is the later risk of the metabolic syndrome, or syndrome X (see below).

This trend is a consequence of the ready availability of highly calorific foods, often with too large a proportion of calories derived from fat. There is much food advertising directed at children and coupled to promotional toys. At the same time there has been a decrease in physical activity because of lack of opportunity to exercise at school and increased sedentary behaviour at home, such as watching television. Thus there is a spiral of decreased fitness, poor body image and increasing weight gain.

In the adult population the differentiation between endocrine and nutritional obesity can be difficult, as obese individuals may have many features of mild Cushing's syndrome (red face, hypertension, glycosuria and raised urinary steroid excretion), and borderline hypothyroidism is quite common. However, in children the distinction is usually clear. Food acts as a fuel for growth, and there is a raised level of insulin and insulin-like growth factor 1 (IGF-1) in the blood. This promotes linear growth, so the child is often relatively tall for their genetic background (see Figure 8.1).

Fat secretes a peptide hormone, leptin, to signal adequate fat stores and regulate food-seeking behaviour (see Figure 8.2).

Leptin also acts to promote cyclical secretion of LH and FSH, thus initiating puberty once a certain fat weight has been achieved. In turn this means that the obese, tall child often goes through an early puberty and growth spurt and has only a modestly elevated final height. As discussed previously (see Chapter 4), a *short* fat child should always prompt concern about an underlying endocrine abnormality.

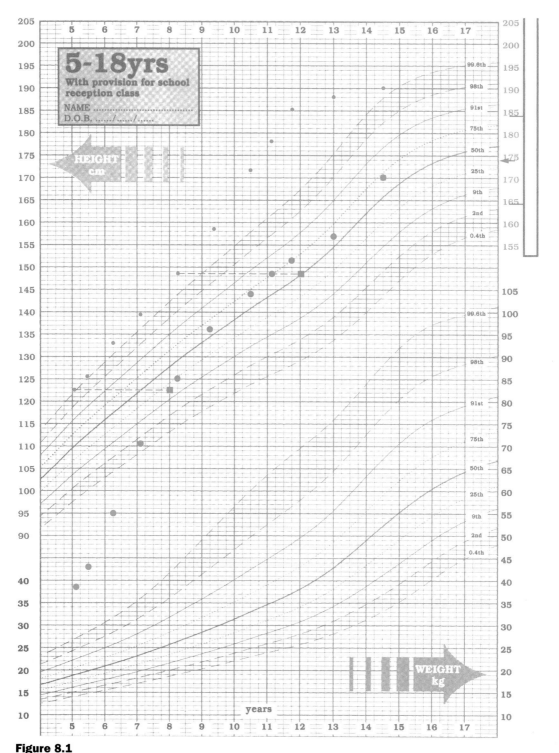

Figure 8.1

Severe nutritional obesity. At presentation at the age of 5.2 years, this child had the approximate weight of a tall 9-year-old, and moderately advanced bone age (8 years). There was no response to diet or family therapy. There were 4 mL testes at 9.5 years, with 12 mL testes and stage 3 pubic hair and penis at 11.2 years. Final height was 6 cm above the target centile range.

A few families and individuals have very rarely been described with a congenital abnormality in leptin secretion or in the receptors and post-receptor mechanisms of the hypothalamus.

Factors that increase the likelihood of genetic defect causing obesity include the following:

- consanguinity;
- family history;
- early-onset severe obesity;
- abnormal food-seeking behaviour;
- hypogonadism;
- red hair (related to dual deficiencies of pigment regulation and appetite suppression, POMC; see Figure 8.2).

Some of these conditions may respond to treatment with biosynthetic leptin. However, the vast majority of obese individuals have high leptin

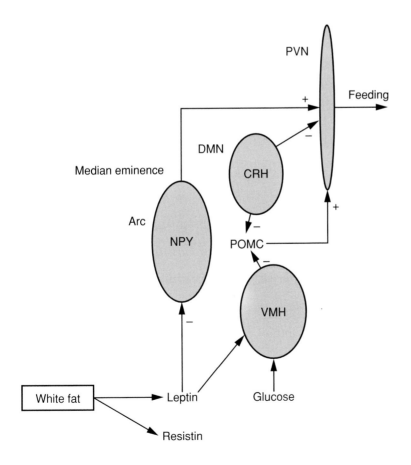

Figure 8.2
Leptin is a peptide hormone secreted by white fat. It circulates and is actively transported across the blood–brain barrier to act on specific receptors in the hypothalamus (ventromedial nucleus, VMN), probably together with other signals from glucose and insulin. Subsequent interactions with neuropeptides (e.g. NPY) and corticotropin-releasing hormone (CRH) and pro-opiomelanocortin (POMC) in the arcuate (Arc) and dorsomedial nucleus (DMN) act to control feeding behaviour mediated through the paraventricular nucleus (PVN). White fat also secretes a newly discovered hormone, resistin, that acts to modify insulin sensitivity in the periphery, which may also modify satiety.

levels in direct relation to their high fat mass, and need more conventional treatment to stabilize their weight. The use of exogenous leptin as a therapy in adult simple obesity has yielded disappointing results.

Work-up of childhood obesity

HISTORY

- Dietary history – *be specific, not general,* and it is important to be non-accusatory (e.g. 'what did he or she eat and drink for breakfast *yesterday,* then snack, then lunch, then snack on the way home from school, etc., including specific amounts of food, type of milk/pop, how many packets of crisps as 'extras', etc.).
- Activity – again be specific with regard to amount, time, 'quality' and frequency. If resources permit, a food/activity diary may be analysed over a 3-day period that includes a weekend day.
- Ask about abnormal behaviour related to food (this may reveal a hypothalamic problem).
- Ask about headaches or symptoms that might suggest a rare intracranial lesion, and enquire about previous CNS insults/trauma that may have damaged the hypothalamus.
- Ask about body image, teasing, showers at school, etc.

EXAMINATION

- Measurement of height, weight and parental height/weight.
- Calculation of body mass index (weight (kg)/height (metres)^2).
- Plotting of BMI on UK centile chart.
- If available, skinfold thickness and calculation of total body fat mass.
- Look for possible hypothyroidism – goitre, dry skin/hair, pale complexion, frontal balding, homonymous hemianopia (hypertrophied TSH-secreting pituitary may compress the optic chiasm), slow reflexes.
- Look for possible Cushing's syndrome (*very rare* except secondary to steroid medication) – thin limbs, centripetal obesity, buffalo hump, striae, hirsutism, hypertension, glycosuria.
- Look for signs of hypothalamic damage (previous brain tumour, irradiation, injury).
- Prader–Willi syndrome – typical face, small hands and feet, learning difficulties, early hypotonia; other rare syndromes of hypothalamic obesity and dysmorphic features.

Look for the following as a consequence of the obesity:

● glycosuria;
● acanthosis nigricans (insulin resistance);
● hirsutism/virilization (PCO);
● hypertension;
● hyperlipidaemia;
● cor pulmonale (shortness of breath, snoring, apnoea);
● orthopaedic problems (bow legs, slipped epiphyses).

Treatment of childhood obesity

In the absence of a rare cause of secondary obesity, and in the early stages of treatment of hypothyroidism, it is necessary to restrict the calorie intake estimated as the requirements for *ideal* weight for height.

Weight	Energy requirements	
<10 kg	100 Kcal/kg/day	0.42 MJ/kg/day
10–20 kg	70 Kcal/kg/day	0.29 MJ/kg/day
>20 kg	40 Kcal/kg/day	0.17 MJ/kg/day

Table 8.1
Approximate energy requirements by weight

The metabolic rate of the obese individual is not reduced, as is often thought, but may in fact be higher than average. Food is needed for growth, as is an adequate intake of vitamins, protein, etc. However, fat contains twice as many calories per gram as carbohydrate and protein, so restriction of calorie intake by reduction of fat intake is often the easiest way to promote weight loss. It is important to seek paediatric dietetic advice in order to ensure adequate and safe nutritional intake during the dieting process.

If a previous weight is known, then the excess weight gained since the last measurement can be calculated as shown in Figure 8.3.

Growing children have the advantage that they can 'grow into' their weight (see Figure 8.3). This may be demonstrated by a steadily decreasing BMI centile. They only need an active weight-reducing diet if they are approaching bony fusion in late puberty or in extreme circumstances (secondary type 2 diabetes, cor pulmonale, immobility, etc.). Weight reduction in infancy should only be attempted in specialist centres. It is probably safest to try to maintain the BMI percentile, or to reduce it very slowly in a growing child.

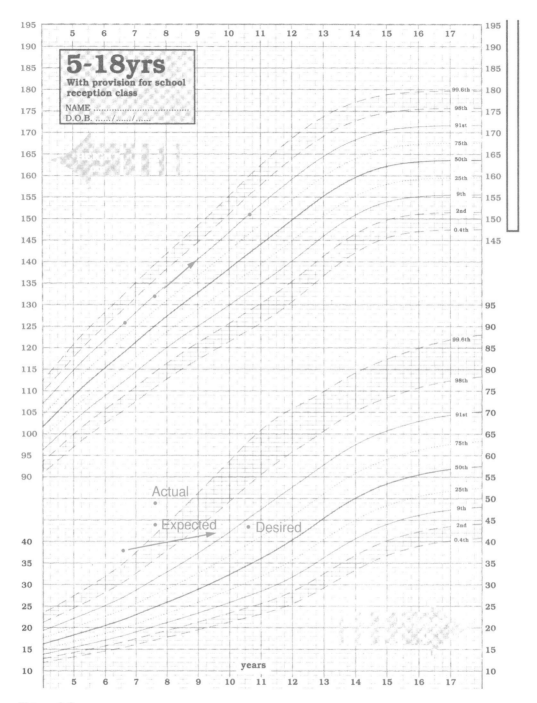

Figure 8.3

Over a 1-year period, the total weight gain is 10.5 kg. If it is gained at the same rate as growth in height, the expected weight gain is 5.5 kg. Therefore the excess gain is 5 kg. The weight will be almost entirely fatty tissue. As 1 kg of fat releases about 7000 Kcal (29 MJ) of energy, 5 kg × 7000 Kcal is equivalent to 35 000 Kcal excess intake in the year, or about 100 Kcal/day. Therefore to reduce the rate of weight gain, one must reduce daily intake by about twice this amount (i.e. 200 Kcal – or less than one packet of crisps) or increase daily activity to consume this amount (equivalent to running about ¾ mile). If maintained, this would put height/weight on the same desired centile after about 3 years.

Coupled with calorie restriction there needs to be active participation in a structured programme of increasing activity and often behaviour modification therapy (usually as a family), overseen by a multidisciplinary team with an interest in the problem. Several studies have shown that frequent supervision and feedback increase the likelihood of success.

By adopting these measures it is possible to achieve normalization of the BMI without subsequent weight gain in *some* well-motivated and well-supported children. Sadly, defaulting on the programme is common especially if there is a family-wide problem with eating.

There are currently no medical therapies that have been licensed or shown to be of benefit in childhood obesity.

Consequences of childhood obesity

The metabolic syndrome, syndrome X, is starting to appear in the childhood population.

It is especially prevalent in areas of economic hardship and in some racial groups (Asian and Afro-Caribbean). It is characterized by hypertension, hyperlipidaemia and insulin resistance with acanthosis. There may be frank type 2 diabetes that requires treatment with oral hypoglycaemic agents in specialized units.

Many girls with obesity show additional evidence of hyperandrogenization. This often presents in late childhood with sweaty armpits, smelly feet, moodiness and acne. True puberty occurs relatively early on, but the signs of excess testosterone production persist, giving rise to increasing cosmetic concern. After menarche, periods may be heavy and painful. This merges into the familiar polycystic ovarian syndrome of adulthood.

Severe obesity, especially in early childhood, may result in shortness of breath on exertion, and periods of snoring and central apnoea at night. There may be frank right-sided cardiac enlargement with cor pulmonale. Non-alcoholic steatohepatitis (NASH) may cause progressive liver function abnormalities and pseudotumour cerebri may cause headaches.

Orthopaedic problems may occur. Slipped upper femoral epiphysis is the commonest abnormality (and if associated with short stature should prompt a search for hypothyroidism and GHD). Some children develop a bowing of the legs to allow locomotion, or may even be restricted to a wheelchair.

Although its incidence is increasing, moderate obesity gives rise to problems of self-image in a world that is paradoxically obsessed with thinness. Children may be teased (to the extent that they may avoid showering at school), and eat for comfort, thus increasing the spiral of further weight gain.

Further reading

University of York NHS Centre for Reviews and Dissemination (1997) *CRD 10 – systematic review of interventions in the treatment and prevention of obesity.* York Publishing Services, York.

Failure to thrive (FTT)

Failure to thrive (FTT) is a label rather than a diagnosis. It describes the common situation of a child in the first 2 years of life who is not gaining weight at an adequate rate. Many definitions of FTT have been suggested that are useful for research purposes and screening programmes, and which are based on the following:

1 centile channel crossing, which depends on the standards used (e.g. the multichannel Sheffield Weight Chart). This can be refined by defining FTT as a loss of more than 1.3 SD (two major centile lines on the current UK charts) from the peak weight centile achieved at 4–8 weeks of age;
2 indices of weight gain related to expected weight velocity (e.g. the 'thrive index' which compares a child's attained and predicted weight SDS using observational data adjusted to allow for regression to the mean and normal variations in weight gain);
3 charts that allow for normal regression to the mean and variations in weight gain (e.g. the Cole chart shown in Figure 9.1, or the Newcastle chart derived from the same data that are used to calculate the thrive index described above).

Different methods vary in their sensitivity and specificity at different ages, so it is important that each unit has its own standard approach to defining the problem, with appropriate local referral guidelines.

In practice, however, the referral is often made on the basis of parental or health visitor concern about the adequacy of weight gain of an infant. Some basic principles should be remembered before referral or investigation is considered.

● Children normally grow in fits and starts, so frequent weighing will produce periods of zero weight gain, or even brief weight loss, in *normal* children. Therefore a reasonable time period should be allowed to elapse between each measurement (at least 1 month).
● Small children are born to small parents. If the length of the child is not taken into account, and if only single measurements of weight are

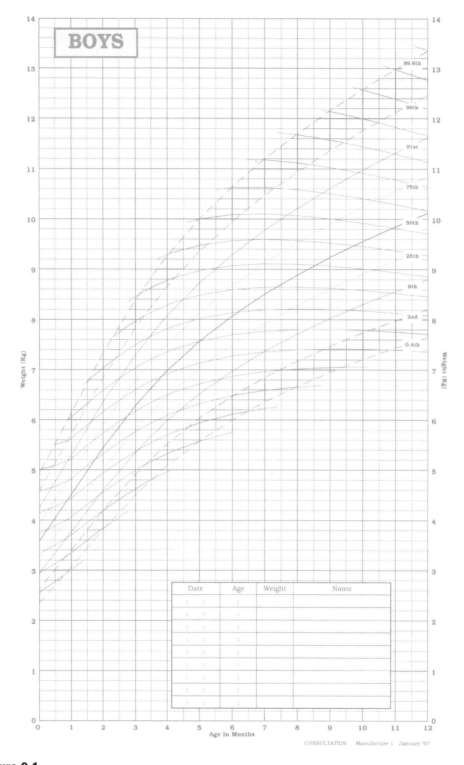

(a)

CONSULTATION   Manufacture 1   January '97

Figure 9.1

Cole 'thrive' chart for (a) boys and (b) girls. The 'thrive lines' are available as an acetate overlay for the hand-held child health record infancy weight charts (see Appendix).

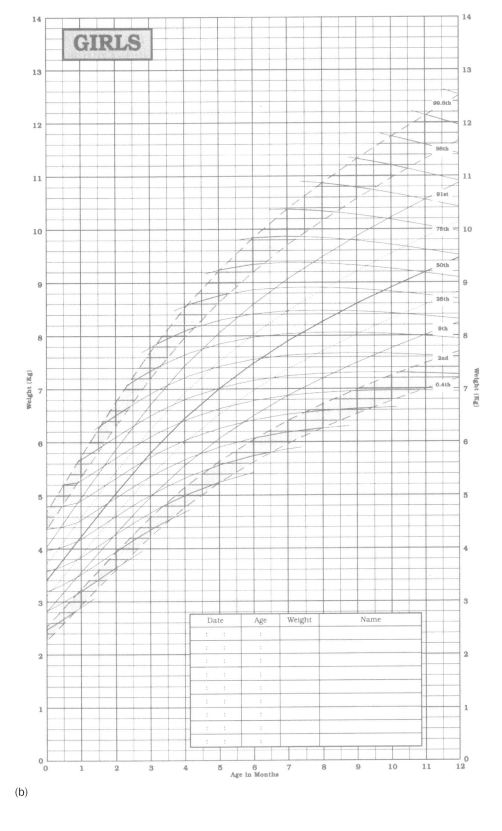

(b)

Figure 9.1 continued

giardia cysts – giardiasis;

fat globules – giardiasis, cystic fibrosis;

enteropathogenic *E.coli* – overgrowth is an uncommon cause of mal-absorption.

- Reducing substances are positive in lactose intolerance – usually post-gastroenteritis, but also associated with severe congenital alactasia (rare) and hypolactasia (common in non-Caucasians). There are other rare disaccharide intolerances (e.g. amaltasia, asucrasia).
- Stool pH is often reduced in the presence of bacterial fermentation of undigested sugars.

URINE

- MC & S – unrecognized urinary tract infections and even renal failure (e.g. due to posterior urethral valves) can cause FTT.
- Reducing substances – diabetes usually presents in older children with polyuria, polydipsia and weight loss. However, it can present in infancy. In individuals with diabetes, glucose (stick) and reducing substances will be positive. Galactosaemia is uncommon, but there will be a negative glucose stick test and positive reducing substances. Further biochemical testing is then indicated.

BLOOD TESTS

- Full blood count – for haemoglobin and mean corpuscular volume in particular. Microcytic anaemia may be secondary to inadequate iron intake, microscopic blood loss (e.g. from coeliac disease and cow's-milk protein intolerance) and is present in renal failure and chronic ill health. Macrocytic anaemia may be secondary to vitamin B_{12} or folate mal-absorption with steatorrhea.
- U&E and creatinine – to exclude hidden renal failure and rare metabolic disorders that cause FTT (e.g. Bartter's syndrome of hyperchloraemic alkalosis).

After these tests, further investigations may be indicated, depending on the results. These investigations are as follows:

- jejunal biopsy (coeliac disease, cow's-milk protein intolerance, disaccharide intolerances);
- sweat tests/immunoreactive trypsin genetic tests for cystic fibrosis;

- chromosomes if there are any dysmorphic features (ring chromosome abnormalities have a predisposition to cause FTT, sometimes with relatively mild dysmorphic features);
- organic and amino acids;
- other metabolic tests.

Diagnosis	Treatment
Cow's milk protein intolerance	Cow's-milk protein-free diet
Coeliac disease	Gluten-free diet
Lactose intolerance	Lactose-free diet
Urinary tract infection	Initial antibiotics, then prophylaxis and investigation of renal tract

Table 9.1
Treatment of some of the commoner diagnosed disorders that cause FTT (usually undertaken in specialist centres)

Further reading

Bisset WM (1998) Disorders of the alimentary tract and liver. In Campbell AGM and McIntosh N (eds), *Textbook of paediatrics*, 5th edn. Churchill Livingstone, Edinburgh, 465–8.

Appendix

Equipment

Charts, thrive-line overlay acetates and growth calculators based on UK 1995 reference figures are available from:
Harlow Printing, Maxwell Street, South Shield NE33 4PU, UK.
Tel: +44 (0) 191 455 4286.
Fax: +44 (0) 191 427 0195.
Email: Sales@harlowprinting.co.uk
Website: www.harlowprinting.co.uk

Down's and Turner Syndrome Charts; charts for leg length, height velocity and skinfold thickness are available from: Castlemead Publications, 12 Little Mundells, Welwyn Garden City, Hertfordshire AL7 1EW

EQUIPMENT SUPPLIERS AND APPROXIMATE COSTS

Please check with suppliers for current price list.

Holtain
Holtain Ltd, Crosswell, Crymych SA41 3UF, UK.
Tel: +44 (0) 1239 891656. Fax: +44 (0) 1239 891453.
Email: holtain@themail.co.uk
Website: http://www.fullbore.co.uk/holtain/medical/welcome.html

Stadiometer with standard counter	£899.00
Infantometer	£555.00
Skinfold calliper	£176.00
Pocket stadiometers	£42.00
Body composition analyser	£1430.00
Body composition analysis software for Windows	£32.00

Child Growth Foundation

Head circumference:

Reusable Lasso-o™ head circumference tapes (pack of 10)	£7

Length:

Pedobaby 2 length measurer (incubator) 0–50 cm	£38.00
Measure mat (infant) 0–92 cm	£23.50
Rollameter (infant) 0–1 m	£59.50
Kiddimeter (infant) 0–1 m	£339.50

Height:

Mimimeter (0–1.83 m)	£29.50
Minimeter (0–2 m)	£30.50
Magnimeter	£246.75
Leicester height measure	£52.00
1-m calibration rod	£10.00

Weight:

Seca 835 3-in-1 (0–14 kg; 0–100 kg; 0–136 kg)	£237.35
Tanita scales (standing) 0–136 kg	£76.50
Weylux 90 (sitting) 0–160 kg	£752.00

Other:

Prader orchidometer	£28.50

Training

The Child Growth Foundation organizes local one-day courses for primary care practitioners, school nurses, community physicians and health visitors. Contact: The Child Growth Foundation, 2 Mayfield Avenue, Chiswick, London W4 1PW, UK.
Tel: 020 8995 0257 or 020 8994 7625.
Email: CGFLondon@aol.com.

One-hour update	£85
Half day	£350
Full day	£475

The Sheffield Neonatal and Children's Auxology 2-day course is held every other year in Sheffield, and the approximate cost is £75. It is intended for advanced training of interested endocrine nurses and physicians, neonatologists and midwives, and involves training in auxological techniques,

including bone age, with supporting lectures and practical classes. Contact
J.K. Wales j.k.wales@sheffield.ac.uk

UK support groups

GENERAL

The Child Growth Foundation, 2 Mayfield Avenue, Chiswick, London
W4 1PW, UK.
Tel: 020 8995 0257 or 020 8994 7625.
Email: CGFLondon@aol.com.

Blanket organization for families and individuals, that includes sections for
short stature, pituitary hormone deficiency, premature sexual maturation,
Turner's and Noonan's syndrome, IUGR and Russell–Silver syndrome.
There are regular newsletters and meetings.

SHORT STATURE

Restricted Growth Association, PO Box 8, Countesthorpe, Leicester
LE8 5ZS, UK.
Tel: 0116 247 8913.
Email: honour@webleicester.co.uk
For children and parents with short stature.

SPECIFIC SYNDROMES

Turner Syndrome Support Society, 1/8 Irving Court, Hardgate, Clydebank
G81 6BA, UK.
Tel: 01389 390385 or 01389 872511.
Email: TurnerSynd@aol.com
Website: http://www.tss.org.uk

OTHER SYNDROMES AND DISORDERS

Contact a Family, 170 Tottenham Court Road, London W1P 0HA, UK.
Tel: 020 7383 3555.
Email: info@cafamily.org.uk

Birth Defects Foundation, Martindale, Hawks Green, Cannock, WS11 2XN, UK.
Tel: 08700 707020.

TALL STATURE

Marfan Association UK, Rochester House, 5 Aldershot Road, Fleet GU13 9NG, UK.
Tel: 01252 810472.
Email: marfan@thenet.co.uk

Klinefelter Syndrome, 56 Little Yeldham Road, Little Yeldham, Halstead CO9 4QT, UK.
Tel: 01787 237460.

Tall Persons' Club GB and Ireland, 29 Stanhope Street, Hereford HR4 0HA, UK.
Tel: 01432 271818.

Sotos' Syndrome, c/o The Child Growth Foundation (see above).

Useful websites

GROWTH CHARTS ON THE INTERNET

Ray Williams Paediatric Endocrine Centre, Sydney, Australia. Includes anthropometric standards, guidelines and texts. http://www.rwi.edu.au/

Downloadable current NCHS US charts. http://www.cdc.gov/growthcharts

Downloadable Down's growth charts. http://www.growthcharts.com

WHO growth charts and database. http://www.who.ch/whosis/cgrowth/cgrowth.html

INTERNATIONAL ENDOCRINE RESOURCES ON THE INTERNET

British Society for Paediatric Endocrinology and Diabetes (BSPED) (professional group). http://bspe.shef.ac.uk

European Society for Paediatric Endocrinology (ESPE) (professional group). http://espe.shef.ac.uk

Lawson Wilkins Society (US paediatric endocrinology professional site). http://lwpes.org/ LWPES

Online Mendelian Inheritance in Man (OMIM), the major reference for all genetic and syndromic disorders. http://www3.ncbi.nlm.nih.gov/omim/

The Diabetes Insipidus Foundation and Support Group. http://diabetes insipidus.maxinter.net

Patient and family information from John Hopkins on congenital adrenal hyperplasia. http://www.med.jhu.edu/pedendo/cah/

Learning about growth: a Serono-sponsored patient information site. http://www.learningaboutgrowth.com

XYXO, Mixed Gonadal Dysgenesis Support Group. http://www.xyxo.org

Yahoo site that provides links to large numbers of sites detailing various medical conditions and information about contacting support groups. http://www.yahoo.co.uk/Health/Diseases_and_Conditions/

NIH rare diseases index. This is another site that lists links to groups providing information on a huge number of rare disorders. http://cancer net.nci.nih.gov/ord/

Noonan's syndrome support. http://www.geocities.com/~noonansyndrome/

The anthropometric desk reference, which includes anthropometric tutorials. http://www.odc.com/anthro/deskref/desktoc.html

Society for the Study of Inborn Errors of Metabolism. http://www.ssiem.org.uk/

ENDO Direct, a website which provides information on new developments in endocrinology. http://www.endo-direct.com

A free resource containing endocrine clinical and pathological images for teaching purposes. http://www.bg.ic.ac.uk/sdg/EndoPics

Index

Page numbers in **bold** type refer to figures; those in *italic* refer to tables or boxed material